Study Guide for

The Human Body in Health and Illness

Third Edition

Barbara Herlihy, PhD, RN
Professor
University of the Incarnate Word
School of Nursing and Health Professions
San Antonio, Texas

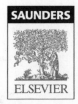

SAUNDERS

ELSEVIER

SAUNDERS
ELSEVIER

11830 Westline Industrial Drive
St. Louis, Missouri 63146

STUDY GUIDE FOR THE HUMAN BODY IN HEALTH AND ILLNESS

ISBN-13: 978-1-4160-2884-0
ISBN-10: 1-4160-2884-6

ISBN-13: 978-1-4160-2884-0
ISBN-10: 1-4160-2884-6

Managing Editor: Jeff Downing
Developmental Editor: Allison M. Brock
Project Manager: Katherine Hinkebein
Cover Designer: Paula Ruckenbrod

Printed in the United States of America

Last digit is the print number: 9   8   7   6   5   4   3

To my students at the University of the Incarnate Word for the millions of questions you have answered over the years and, most importantly, for your warmth, affection, and friendship.

Barbara Herlihy

Preface

Questions, questions, and more questions! The *Study Guide for The Human Body in Health and Illness* is designed to help you to learn the basic concepts of anatomy and physiology through relentless questioning. Each chapter in the *Study Guide* corresponds to a chapter in the textbook. Some questions are easy and require simple recall; other exercises are more difficult and are designed to help you synthesize and integrate basic concepts. A strategy that I have found very helpful is to ask the same question in several different ways. This strategy requires you to view the content from several different perspectives and encourages you to think critically through and integrate many seemingly unrelated facts. This *Study Guide* will make you work.

It is recommended that you work through all the exercises in every chapter. Working in groups reduces stress, encourages learning, and makes the learning process more enjoyable. More importantly, student-to-student interaction encourages active learning.

ORGANIZATION

The *Study Guide* chapters are divided into three parts: **Part I, Mastering the Basics**, contains matching, ordering, labeling, diagram reading, and coloring exercises for each content area in the corresponding textbook chapter. These exercises help you learn basic anatomy and physiology knowledge; **Part II, Putting It All Together**, contains multiple-choice practice quizzes and case studies that integrate the chapter content; and **Part III, Challenge Yourself!**, contains grouping exercises and word puzzles.

Throughout the *Study Guide*, there is a concerted effort to use the medical terminology that was introduced in the textbook and will certainly be used in clinical situations. For instance, words such as *diagnosis, hypokalemia,* and *hyperglycemia* are used frequently and require mastery. As in the textbook, *pathophysiology* is used when it serves to explain the normal anatomy and physiology.

Throughout the *Study Guide*, page references from the textbook are provided to assist you in answering the questions. A complete Answer Key has been provided for your instructor.

PART I: MASTERING THE BASICS

Matching

You are asked to match the words or terms in one column with descriptive terms in a second column.

Ordering

The ordering exercises ask you to arrange a series of events or structures in the correct order. For instance, one exercise is ordering the structures through which blood flows from the right atrium through the heart to the aorta. Other ordering exercises include the sequence of events at the neuromuscular junction, the flow of urine from the kidney through the urethra, and the flow of blood from the finger to the toe.

Labeling and Coloring

Many of the illustrations that appear in the textbook are reproduced in the *Study Guide*. You will need to label the figure and, in some instances, color a particular part of it. Coloring helps to focus your attention on a particularly important anatomic structure. For example, color the right side of the heart blue, indicating unoxygenated blood, and the left side red, indicating oxygenated blood.

For more coloring activities, see the *Body Spectrum* CD-ROM provided free with your textbook.

Read the Diagram

These exercises ask you to interpret illustrations from the textbook to promote understanding of a particular function or process.

PART II: PUTTING IT ALL TOGETHER

Multiple-Choice Questions

Each chapter contains multiple-choice questions. In addition, a simple case study and a series of related multiple-choice questions appear at the end of each chapter.

PART III: CHALLENGE YOURSELF!

Groups and Puzzles

Part III includes Groups and Puzzles. The grouping exercise asks you to integrate information by grouping together related topics and excluding unrelated topics. The puzzles, while entertaining, are integrative and instructive. You are asked to eliminate anatomical terms until you discover the answer. A hint appears in the title.

Acknowledgments

As with the text, the creation and publication of this *Study Guide* involved the combined efforts of many people. I want to thank the staff of Elsevier Science for their efforts; they are talented, beyond competent, and just plain nice. I especially want to thank Allison Brock for her encouragement, persistence, patience, sense of humor, and close attention to detail.

Many thanks to my family: Jerry, Kellie, Joey, and Kristan, for enduring another edition. Same to the pet population, which faithfully camped out around my cluttered writing table.

Contents

Introduction to the Human Body

Answer Key: Textbook page references are provided as a guide for answering these questions. A complete answer key was provided for your instructor.

Objectives

1. Define the terms anatomy and physiology.

2. List the levels of organization of the human body.

3. Describe the 11 major organ systems.

4. Define homeostasis.

5. Describe the anatomical position.

6. List common terms used for relative positions of the body.

7. Describe the three major planes of the body.

8. List anatomical terms for regions of the body.

9. Describe the major cavities of the body.

PART I: MASTERING THE BASICS

MATCHING

General Terms

Directions. Match the following terms to the most appropriate definition by writing the correct letter in the space provided. Some terms may be used more than once. See text pp. 2-6.

A. physiology

B. homeostasis

C. pathophysiology

D. anatomy

1. __D__ branch of science that studies the structure of the body

2. __A__ branch of science that describes how the body functions

3. __C__ branch of science that describes the consequences of improper function of the body (as in disease)

4. __D__ word from the Greek meaning "to dissect"

5. __B__ word describing, for example, body temperature remaining at 37°C (98.6°F), despite the fact that the person is swimming in water that is 22°C (72°F)

6. __B__ word describing the lowering of blood glucose to normal after eating a meal

Student Name _____

MATCHING

Anatomical Terms

Directions. Match the following terms to the most appropriate definition by writing the correct letter in the space provided. Some terms may be used more than once. See text p. 7.

A. superior	E. proximal	I. lateral
B. medial	F. superficial	J. posterior
C. distal	G. anterior	K. deep
D. inferior	H. anatomical position	L. peripheral

1. **H** the body is standing erect, with the face forward, the arms at the side, and the toes and the palms of the hands directed forward

2. **A** part that is above another part or is closer to the head; opposite of *inferior*

3. **G** toward the front (the belly surface); another word is *ventral*

4. **J** toward the back surface; another word is *dorsal*

5. **D** part that is located below another part or is closer to the feet; opposite of *superior*

6. **B** toward the midline of the body; opposite of *lateral*

7. **E** structure that is nearer the trunk or main part of the body; opposite of *distal*

8. **F** part that is located on or near the surface of the body; opposite of *deep*

9. **L** part that is located away from the center; opposite of *central*

10. **I** away from the midline of the body; opposite of *medial*

11. **L** position of the blood vessels relative to the heart (central location)

12. **K** opposite of *superficial*

13. **C** opposite of *proximal*

READ THE DIAGRAM

Directions. Referring to the diagram, fill in the spaces with the correct letters. Not all letters are used [(L) is left; (R) is right]. See text pp. 7-9.

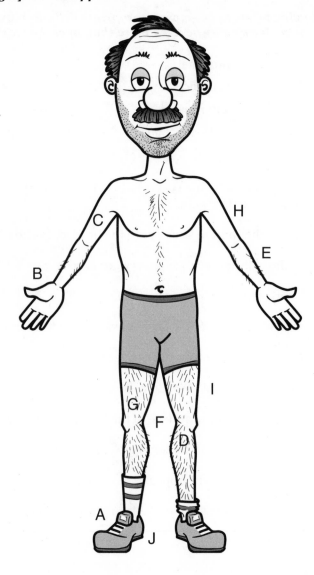

1. __E__   point that is distal to the (L) elbow and proximal to the wrist

2. __C__   point that is immediately proximal to the (R) elbow

3. __D__   point that is immediately distal to the (L) patella

4. __G__   point that is immediately proximal to the (R) patella

5. __A__   point that indicates the lateral aspect of the (R) foot

6. __I__   point that is distal to the (L) hip and proximal to the knee

7. __J__   point that indicates the medial aspect of the right foot

8. __H__   point that is distal to the (L) axillary area and proximal to the antecubital area

Student Name _____

Xs, Ys, Zs, AND CIRCLES

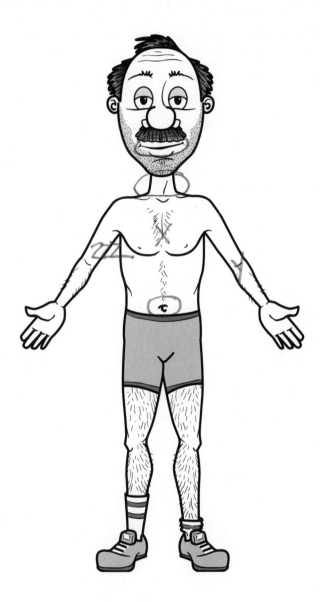

1. Encircle the following areas: cervical, oral, umbilical.

2. Place a string of Xs along the sternal area.

3. Place Ys in the antecubital spaces.

4. Place a string of Zs along the brachial areas.

MATCHING

Regional Body Terms

Directions. Match the following terms to the most appropriate definition by writing the correct letter in the space provided. See text pp. 8-9.

A. digital
B. axillary
C. buccal
D. cervical
E. lumbar
F. deltoid
G. scapular

H. umbilical
I. antecubital
J. gluteal
K. inguinal
L. oral
M. occipital
N. pubic

O. patellar
P. pedal
Q. popliteal
R. femoral
S. brachial
T. sternal
U. flank

1. __D__   neck region

2. __K__   groin region

3. __H__   navel or "belly button" area

4. __B__   armpit

5. __O__   kneecap area

6. __C__   between the cheek and gum

7. __L__   pertaining to the mouth

8. __M__   pertaining to the back (posterior) of the head

9. __E__   lower back area, extending from the chest to the hips

10. __J__   where you sit; the buttocks area

11. __I__   front aspect of the elbow area

12. __Q__   area behind the knee

13. __F__   shoulder area

14. __T__   breastbone area

15. __N__   genital area

16. __S__   referring to the arm

17. __A__   referring to fingers and toes

18. __P__   foot area

19. __G__   shoulder blade area

20. __U__   area on the sides between the lower ribs and hip

21. __R__   thigh region

Student Name _____

MATCHING

Cavities of the Body

Directions. Match the following terms to the most appropriate definition by writing the correct letter in the space provided. Some terms may be used more than once. See text pp. 9-12.

A. dorsal cavity
B. cranial cavity
C. vertebral canal (cavity)

D. thoracic cavity
E. ventral cavity

F. abdominopelvic cavity
G. pleural cavity

1. __B__   cavity that is located in the skull and contains the brain

2. __C__   cavity that extends from the cranial cavity; it contains the spinal cord

3. __C__   also called the *spinal canal*

4. __E__   cavity that is located in the front of the body; it contains the thoracic cavity and the abdominopelvic cavity

5. __F__   cavity that is divided into quadrants

6. __A__   cavity that is located toward the back of the body; contains the cranial cavity and the vertebral canal

7. __D__   upper ventral cavity that is surrounded by ribs; is largely filled with the lungs and contains the mediastinum

8. __F__   lower ventral cavity that is separated from the thoracic cavity by the diaphragm

9. __D__   part of the ventral cavity that contains the mediastinum

10. __G__   part of the thoracic cavity that contains the lungs

READ THE DIAGRAM

Directions. Indicate the letter on the diagram that is described below. ([L] is left; [R] is right). Not all letters are used. Some letters may be used more than once.

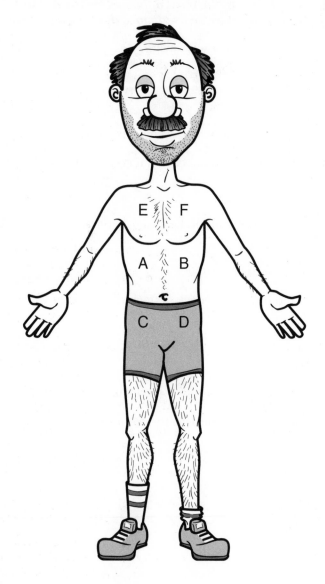

1. __D__ the point that is inferior to the diaphragm and is located in the left lower quadrant (LLQ)

2. __F__ the point over the left pleural cavity

3. __A__ the point that is in both the right upper quadrant (RUQ) and (R) hypochondriac region

4. __A__ the point on the right side of the body that is superior to the umbilicus and inferior to the diaphragm

5. __C__ the point of pain for acute appendicitis; right lower quadrant (RLQ)

Student Name _____

PART II: PUTTING IT ALL TOGETHER

MULTIPLE CHOICE

Directions. Choose the correct answer.

1. The heart and blood vessels work together to pump blood throughout the body. What is the word that describes the heart and blood vessels?

    a. tissue
    b. molecule
    c. organ
    d. organ system

2. The inguinal region

    a. is in the thoracic cavity.
    b. houses the heart.
    c. refers to the groin.
    d. is superior to the umbilical region.

3. The sternum (breastbone) is

    a. inferior to the umbilicus.
    b. deep to the lungs.
    c. superficial to the heart.
    d. posterior to the heart.

4. Which word describes the route of administration of a drug given by mouth?

    a. cranial
    b. inguinal
    c. oral
    d. antecubital

5. The appendix is located in the RLQ of which cavity?

    a. dorsal
    b. cranial
    c. abdominopelvic
    d. spinal

6. The liver is located in the RUQ and the appendix is located in the RLQ. Which of the following describes the position of the liver relative to the appendix?

    a. distal
    b. superior
    c. anterior
    d. deep

7. Which region surrounds the navel (belly button)?

    a. epigastric region
    b. popliteal area
    c. umbilical region
    d. right iliac region

8. Which of the following regions is included within the RUQ?

    a. umbilical
    b. hypogastric
    c. right iliac
    d. right hypochondriac

9. Which of the following describes the division of the body by a transverse plane?

    a. a front and a back
    b. a left and a right
    c. a top and a bottom
    d. an inside and an outside

10. Which of the following describes the division of the body by a coronal plane?

    a. a front and a back
    b. a top and a bottom
    c. a left and a right
    d. an inside and an outside

11. Which of the following describes the division of the body by a sagittal plane?

    a. a front and a back
    b. a left and a right
    c. a top and a bottom
    d. an inside and an outside

12. Which of the following describes the division of the body into a front and back?

    a. the frontal plane
    b. the sagittal plane
    c. a cross section
    d. transverse plane

13. Which of the following describes the position of the wrist relative to the elbow?

    a. proximal
    b. superior
    c. dorsal
    d. distal ✓

14. Which of the following describes the position of the antecubital space relative to the carpal region?

    a. proximal ✓
    b. medial
    c. distal
    d. deep

15. Which of the following describes the position of the wrist relative to the fingers?

    a. proximal ✓
    b. inferior
    c. ventral
    d. distal

16. The mediastinum is contained within which cavity?

    a. dorsal
    b. abdominal
    c. pelvic
    d. thoracic ✓

PART III: CHALLENGE YOURSELF!

GROUPS AND PUZZLE

1. Which group is incorrect?

    a. planes: transverse, sagittal, frontal
    b. ventral cavities: thoracic, abdominopelvic, spinal ✓
    c. cavities: dorsal, ventral
    d. organs: heart, stomach, lungs, glands

2. Which group is incorrect?

    a. cavities: dorsal, ventral
    b. ventral cavities: thoracic, abdominopelvic
    c. organ systems: circulatory, digestive, respiratory, immune
    d. organs: heart, stomach, lungs, mediastinum ✓

3. Which group is incorrect?

    a. planes: transverse, sagittal, frontal
    b. cavities: dorsal, ventral
    c. dorsal cavities: thoracic, abdominopelvic ✓
    d. organ systems: skeletal, digestive, respiratory, immune

Student Name _____

PUZZLE

Hint: Navel Gazing Territory

Directions. Perform the following functions on the Sequence of Words below. When all the functions have been performed, you are left with word(s) that are related to the hint. Record your answer below.

Functions: remove the following

1. four quadrants

2. word for the groin area

3. words (3) that refer to parts of the upper extremity

4. words (4) that refer to parts of the lower extremities

5. cavities (3) of the ventral cavity

6. cavities (2) of the dorsal cavity

7. word for the lower back region

8. membranes (2) that have a visceral and parietal layer

9. planes of the body (3)

Sequence of Words

CORONALBRACHIALCRANIALINGUINALLUMBARABDOMINOPELVICTHORACICPERITO
NEUMTRANSVERSEPATELLARRUQDIGITALFEMORALPLEURALUQRLQUMBILICALRE
GIONPEDALANTECUBITALSAGITTALSPINALLLQPLEURALPOPLITEAL

Answer: Umbilical region

BODY TOON

Hint: the type of thinking you need to study anatomy and physiology. (See bottom of page for answer.)

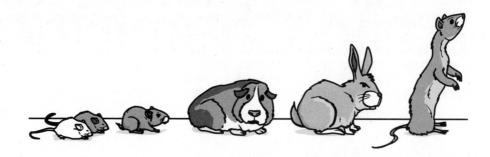

2

Basic Chemistry

Answer Key: Textbook page references are provided as a guide for answering these questions. A complete answer key was provided for your instructor.

Objectives

1. Define the terms matter and element.

2. List the four elements that compose 96% of body weight.

3. Describe the three components of an atom.

4. Describe the role of electrons in the formation of chemical bonds.

5. Differentiate among ionic, covalent, and hydrogen bonds.

6. Explain the differences among electrolytes, ions, cations, and anions.

7. Explain the difference between a molecule and a compound.

8. List five reasons why water is essential to life.

9. Define energy and describe the role of adenosine triphosphate (ATP) in energy transfer.

10. Explain the role of catalysts and enzymes.

11. Differentiate between an acid and a base.

12. Define pH.

13. Differentiate between a mixture, solution, suspension, and colloidal suspension.

PART I: MASTERING THE BASICS

MATCHING

Matter, Elements, and Atoms

Directions. Match the following words and symbols to the most appropriate definition by writing the correct letter in the space provided. Some words and symbols may be used more than once. See text pp. 15-17.

A.	chemistry	E. K	I. O
B.	matter	F. Cl	J. N
C.	element	G. Na	K. H
D.	atom	H. Ca	

1. _____   a fundamental substance that cannot be broken down into a simpler form by ordinary chemical means

2. _____   smallest unit of an element that has that element's characteristics

3. _____   anything that occupies space and has weight

4. _____   composed of millions of identical atoms

5. _____   composed of three particles: protons, neutrons, and electrons

6. _____   exists in three states: solid, liquid, and gas

7. _____   the study of matter

8. _____   symbol for oxygen

9. _____   symbol for sodium

10. _____   symbol for nitrogen

11. _____   symbol for potassium

12. _____   symbol for hydrogen

13. _____   symbol for calcium

14. _____   symbol for chlorine

Student Name _____

MATCHING

The Atom

Directions. Match the following terms to the most appropriate definition by writing the correct letter in the space provided. Some terms may be used more than once. See text pp. 15-17.

A. electron(s)   D. atomic number   G. radioactivity

B. proton   E. atomic weight   H. isotope

C. neutron   F. radioisotope

1. _____   number of protons in the nucleus

2. _____   sum of the protons and the neutrons

3. _____   helium has 2 protons and 2 neutrons; this is what the number 2 indicates

4. _____   helium has 2 protons and 2 neutrons; this is what the number 4 indicates

5. _____   carries a negative charge and circulates in orbits around the nucleus

6. _____   carries a positive charge and is located within the nucleus

7. _____   has a neutral charge and is located within the nucleus

8. _____   in each atom, the number of these is equal to the number of protons

9. _____   different form of the same element (same atomic number but a different atomic weight); an example is "heavy hydrogen"

10. _____   unstable isotope

11. _____   spontaneous decay of a radioisotope

MATCHING

Bonds

Directions. Match the following words to the most appropriate definition by writing the correct letter in the space provided. Some words may be used more than once. See text pp. 17-19.

A.　ionic bond

B.　covalent bond

C.　hydrogen bond

1.　_____　type of bond formed when electrons are shared by atoms

2.　_____　type of bond that forms between water molecules

3.　_____　type of bond that forms water, H_2O

4.　_____　type of bond between sodium and chloride in table salt, NaCl

5.　_____　an intermolecular bond

6.　_____　type of bond formed when one atom donates an electron to another atom

7.　_____　the type of bond usually formed when carbon interacts with another atom

MATCHING

Cations, Anions, Electrolytes

Directions. Match the following words to the most appropriate definition by writing the correct letter in the space provided. Some words may be used more than once. See text pp. 19-20.

A.　cation

B.　anion

C.　electrolyte

D.　ion

E.　ionization

1.　_____　atom that carries an electrical charge

2.　_____　sodium ion

3.　_____　chloride ion

4.　_____　formed as electrons are either lost or gained

5.　_____　classification of NaCl

6.　_____　positively charged ion

7.　_____　negatively charged ion

8.　_____　ion that is represented as Ca^{2+}

9.　_____　dissociation of NaCl into Na^+ and Cl^-

10.　_____　substance that can ionize

Student Name _____

MATCHING

Molecules and Compounds

Directions. Match the following words to the most appropriate definition by writing the correct letter in the space provided. Some words may be used more than once. See text pp. 20-22.

A. water

B. oxygen

C. carbon dioxide

D. chemical reaction

E. catalyst

F. molecule(s)

G. compound(s)

1. _____ O_2 and N_2 are molecules; also classified as _____

2. _____ substances that contain molecules formed by two or more different atoms

3. _____ classification of H_2O, in addition to *molecule*

4. _____ most abundant compound in the body

5. _____ molecule that exists in nature as a gas and plays an essential metabolic role in supplying the cells of the body with energy

6. _____ compound is a waste product that is formed when food is chemically broken down for energy

7. _____ this molecule is the reason why cardiopulmonary resuscitation (CPR) must be started immediately

8. _____ compound that is considered to be the universal solvent

9. _____ compound that has the ability to absorb large amounts of heat without itself increasing dramatically in temperature

10. _____ describes, for example, glucose + O_2 → CO_2 + H_2O + energy

11. _____ describes the role of an enzyme that increases the rate of a chemical reaction

MATCHING

Acids and Bases

Directions. Match the following words and symbols to the most appropriate definition by writing the correct letter in the space provided. Some words and symbols may be used more than once. See text pp. 22-23.

A. acid or acidic

B. base or basic

C. buffer

D. pH

1. _____   a scale, ranging from 0 to 14, that measures how many H^+ are in solution

2. _____   electrolyte that dissociates into H^+ and an anion

3. _____   substance that removes H^+ from solution

4. _____   describes a pH of 7.6

5. _____   describes the effect of an antacid on stomach H^+

6. _____   describes grapefruit juice, vinegar, and lemon juice

7. _____   also referred to as *alkaline*

8. _____   chemical substance that prevents large changes in pH

9. _____   describes normal pH of urine

10. _____   describes normal pH of blood

11. _____   describes normal pH of gastric (stomach) juice

12. _____   substance that can either donate or remove H^+ from solution

READ THE DIAGRAM

pH Scale

Directions. Referring to Figure 2-6 in the textbook, write the numbers from the pH scale in the spaces below. See text pp. 22-23.

1. _____   Which number indicates a neutral pH?

2. _____   What is the acidic range?

3. _____   What is the basic range?

4. _____   What is the alkaline range?

5. _____   Relative to pH 7, which numbers indicate a higher concentration of H^+?

6. _____   Relative to pH 7, which numbers indicate a lower concentration of H^+?

7. _____   Range for blood pH

8. _____   Range for intestinal contents

9. _____   Range for stomach contents

10. _____   Range for urine

Student Name _____

MATCHING

Energy

Directions. Match the following words and symbols to the most appropriate definition by writing the correct letter in the space provided. Some words and symbols may be used more than once. See text pp. 24-25.

A. mechanical   D. chemical   F. radiant

B. thermal   E. electrical   G. ATP

C. nuclear

1. _____ a log is burned, providing light as chemical energy is converted into this type of energy

2. _____ walking is an expression of this type of energy

3. _____ a log is burned, warming everyone around the campfire as chemical energy is converted into this type of energy

4. _____ the heart pushes blood into large blood vessels as chemical energy is converted into this type of energy

5. _____ type of energy that holds atoms together

6. _____ type of energy that is released from the movement of ions

7. _____ energy transfer substance

8. _____ the unstable nucleus of an isotope spontaneously decays, thereby emitting this type of energy

9. _____ responsible for body temperature as chemical energy is converted to this type of energy

MATCHING

Mixtures, Solutions, and Suspensions

Directions. Match the following words to the most appropriate definition by writing the correct letter in the space provided. Some words may be used more than once. See text pp. 25-26.

A. mixture   C. suspension(s)   E. colloidal suspension

B. solution   D. aqueous solution   F. tincture

1. _____ an example is blood plasma because the proteins remain suspended within the plasma

2. _____ solution in which water is the solvent

3. _____ solution in which alcohol is the solvent

4. _____ combinations of two or more substances that can be separated by ordinary physical means

5. _____ examples include mayonnaise, egg white, and jellies

6. _____ mixture that contains a solvent and solute; there is an even distribution of the solute with the solution

7. _____ combination of sugar and little bits of iron

8. _____ an example is sea or salt water

9. _____ mixture that must be shaken to prevent settling of particles

10. _____ suspension in which the particles are so small that they do not need to be shaken to keep them evenly distributed

PART II: PUTTING IT ALL TOGETHER

MULTIPLE CHOICE

Directions. Choose the correct answer.

1. Which of the following describes activities such as chewing food and chopping a log?

    a. chemical change
    b. neutralization reaction
    c. ionization reaction
    d. physical change

2. Which of the following is a strong acid?

    a. vinegar
    b. lemon juice
    c. blood
    d. HCl

3. Which of the following is/are classified as thermal, chemical, and radiant?

    a. cations
    b. anions
    c. energy
    d. electrolytes

Student Name _____

4. Which of the following words best describes a radioisotope?

   a. acidic
   b. alkaline
   c. unstable
   d. ionization

5. Which of the following describes the chlorine atom when its outer electron shell gains one electron?

   a. +1 positive charge
   b. no electrical charge
   c. −2 negative charge
   d. −1 negative charge

6. Hydrogen has 1 proton, 0 neutrons, and 1 electron. Which statement is true?

   a. the atomic number is 2
   b. the atomic weight is 2
   c. the atomic number is 1
   d. this is an isotope of helium because it has no neutrons

7. What type of bond is formed when two hydrogen atoms and one oxygen atom unite to form water?

   a. ionic
   b. hydrogen
   c. intermolecular
   d. covalent

8. What type of reaction occurs when HCl is mixed with a NaOH solution to form a salt (NaCl) and water?

   a. neutralization
   b. agglutination
   c. differentiation
   d. catabolism

9. What is the pH range of blood?

   a. 4.75 to 5.50
   b. 8.45 to 8.95
   c. 7.35 to 7.45
   d. 7.00 to 7.35

10. Which of the following is an electrolyte?

    a. potassium chloride
    b. glucose
    c. water
    d. mayonnaise

11. Which of the following is most acidic?

    a. stomach contents
    b. blood
    c. pH 7.2
    d. urine

12. The sodium ion is a(n)

    a. electrolyte.
    b. anion.
    c. compound.
    d. cation.

13. A blood pH of 7.2

    a. has fewer H^+ than normal blood pH.
    b. is acidosis.
    c. is within normal limits.
    d. is alkalosis.

14. Best described as "very negative."

    a. Al Kaline
    b. Cal Cium
    c. Anne Ion
    d. Hy D. Rogen

PART III: CHALLENGE YOURSELF!

GROUPS AND PUZZLE

1. Which group is incorrect?

    a. parts of an atom: proton, neutron, electron
    b. electrolytes: NaCl, $CaCl_2$, KCl
    c. chemical bonds: ionic, covalent, intermolecular
    d. cations: sodium ion, potassium ion, chloride ion

2. Which group is incorrect?

    a. parts of an atom: proton, neutron, electron
    b. cations: sodium ion, potassium ion, calcium ion
    c. states of matter: solid, liquid, gas
    d. trace elements: copper, calcium, hydrogen

3. Which group is incorrect?

    a. chemical bonds: ionic, covalent, intermolecular
    b. ions: cations, anions
    c. parts of an atom: protons, neutrons, electrons
    d. carriers of a negative charge: electrons, anions, neutrons

BODY TOON

Hint: Spray-painting the town

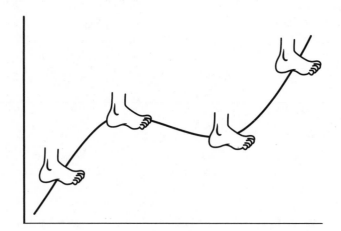

Answer: graph-feetie (graffiti)

Student Name _____

PUZZLE

Hint: YUM....NaCHOs

Directions. Perform the following functions on the Sequence of Words below. When all the functions have been performed, you are left with word(s) that are related to the hint. Record your answer below.

Functions: remove the following

1. clinical condition characterized by a pH of <7.35
2. clinical condition characterized by a pH of >7.45
3. parts (3) of a atom
4. color of an acid on the pH scale
5. color of a base on the pH scale
6. another word for basic
7. types of bonds (2); sharing and donating
8. most prevalent compound in the body
9. energy-transfer molecule
10. name of a water solution and an alcohol solution

Sequence of Words

WATERSODIUMATPALKALINECOVALENTCARBONALKALOSISELECTONSPINKPROTO
NSHYDROGENNEUTRONSAQUEOUSOXYGENIONICBLUEACIDOSISSULFURTINCTURE

Answer: _____

3
Cells

Objectives

1. Label a diagram of the main parts of a typical cell.

2. Describe the functions of the main organelles of the cell.

3. Explain the role of the nucleus.

4. Identify the structure of the cell membrane.

5. Describe the active and passive movement of substances across a cell membrane.

6. Define tonicity and compare isotonic, hypotonic, and hypertonic solutions.

7. Describe the phases of the cell cycle, including mitosis.

8. Explain what is meant by cell differentiation.

PART I: MASTERING THE BASICS

MATCHING

Parts of a Typical Cell

Directions. Match the following terms to the most appropriate definition by writing the correct letter in the space provided. Some terms may be used more than once. See text pp. 30-35.

A. mitochondria	F. lysosomes	K. Golgi apparatus
B. nucleus	G. flagellum	L. rough endoplasmic reticulum (RER)
C. microtubules	H. centrioles	M. smooth endoplasmic reticulum (SER)
D. cilia	I. nuclear membrane	N. cell membrane
E. ribosomes	J. cytoplasm	

1. _____ control center of the cell

2. _____ slipper-shaped organelles that produce most of the energy (ATP)

3. _____ puts the finishing touches on and packages the protein for export from the cell

4. _____ structure that separates the nucleus from the cytoplasm

5. _____ sandpaper-like structure dotted with ribosomes; concerned with protein synthesis

6. _____ long, hairlike projection on the external surface of the cell membrane, such as the tail of the sperm

7. _____ contains most of the DNA

8. _____ selectively permeable structure that separates intracellular material from extracellular material

9. _____ short, hairlike projections on the outer surface of the cell

10. _____ digestive organelles that "clean house" within the cell

11. _____ organelles that help maintain the shape of the cell and assist the cell with movement

12. _____ gel-like substance inside the cell but outside the nucleus

13. _____ organelles that are either bound to the endoplasmic reticulum or are free in the cytoplasm; they are concerned with protein synthesis

14. _____ type of endoplasmic reticulum concerned with the synthesis of lipids and steroids; does not contain ribosomes

15. _____ rod-shaped structures that play a key role in cellular reproduction

16. _____ called the power plants of the cells

Student Name _____

READ THE DIAGRAM

The Typical Cell

Directions. Refer to the diagram and fill in the numbers in the spaces below. See text pp. 30-35.

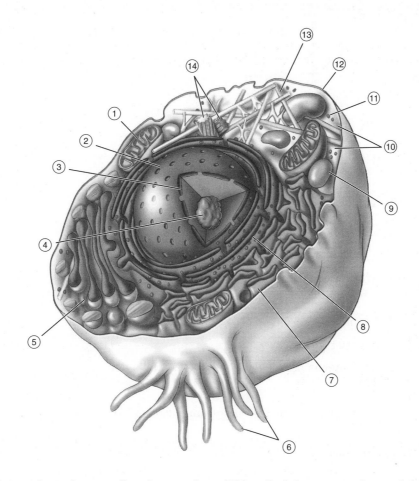

1. _____ slipper-shaped organelles that produce ATP; called the power plants of the cell

2. _____ puts the finishing touches on and packages the protein for export from the cell

3. _____ sandpaper-like structure dotted with ribosomes; concerned with protein synthesis

4. _____ selectively permeable structure that separates intracellular material from extracellular material

5. _____ short, hairlike projections on the outer surface of the cell

6. _____ digestive organelles that "clean house" within the cell

7. _____ organelles that maintain the shape of the cell and assist the cell with movement

8. _____ gel-like substance inside the cell but outside the nucleus

9. _____ type of endoplasmic reticulum concerned with the synthesis of lipids and steroids; does not contain ribosomes

10. _____ rod-shaped structures that play a key role in cellular reproduction

MATCHING

Transport Mechanisms

Directions. Match the following terms to the most appropriate definition by writing the correct letter in the space provided. Some terms may be used more than once. See text pp. 35-40.

A. osmosis   D. phagocytosis   G. pinocytosis

B. diffusion   E. exocytosis   H. filtration

C. facilitated diffusion   F. active transport pump

1. _____ most commonly used transport mechanism

2. _____ transport mechanism in which water diffuses from an area where there is more water to an area where there is less water; the solute cannot diffuse

3. _____ a pressure gradient is the driving force for this type of transport

4. _____ transport mechanism that engulfs a solid particle by the cell membrane; a type of endocytosis

5. _____ transport mechanism that requires an input of energy to move molecules from an area of lesser concentration to an area of greater concentration

6. _____ movement of a substance from an area of higher concentration to an area of lower concentration

7. _____ passive transport mechanism in which glucose is helped across the cell membrane by a helper molecule

8. _____ intake of liquid droplets by the cell membrane; also called *cellular drinking*

9. _____ an example of this transport mechanism is the swelling of a blood clot as water is pulled into the clot

10. _____ describes this type of transport: the blood pressure pushes water and dissolved solute out of the capillaries into the tissue spaces

11. _____ a lysosome eats or ingests a bacterium

12. _____ a protein-containing vesicle within a cell fuses with the cell membrane and ejects the protein

13. _____ transport mechanism that is needed to move additional potassium into the cell if the intracellular concentration of potassium is greater than the extracellular concentration of potassium

Student Name _____

MATCHING

Tonicity

Directions. Match the following terms to the most appropriate definition by writing the correct letter in the space provided. Some terms may be used more than once. See text pp. 38-39.

A. isotonic   C. hemolysis   E. crenation

B. hypotonic   D. hypertonic

1. _____ shrinking of red blood cells

2. _____ bursting of red blood cells

3. _____ solution that is more dilute than the inside of the cell

4. _____ solution with the same concentration as the solution to which it is compared

5. _____ solution that is more concentrated than the inside of the cell

6. _____ a solution that causes crenation of a red blood cell

7. _____ a solution that causes the red blood cell to hemolyze

8. _____ normal saline

9. _____ describes a 10% dextrose solution relative to plasma if a 5% dextrose solution is isotonic to plasma

10. _____ describes pure water relative to plasma

BODY TOON

Hint: enzyme

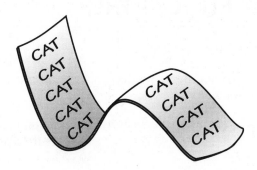

Answer: cat-a-list (catalyst)

MATCHING

Cell Division

Directions. Match the following terms to the most appropriate definition by writing the correct letter in the space provided. See text pp. 41-43.

A. cell cycle

B. cancer

C. mitosis

D. metastasis

E. interphase

F. meiosis

G. G_0

H. stem cell

1. _____ malignant neoplasm

2. _____ ability of cancer cells to spread to distant sites

3. _____ consists of two phases: interphase and mitosis

4. _____ a cell that can specialize into a blood cell, nerve cell, muscle cell, etc.

5. _____ type of cell division involved in bodily growth and repair

6. _____ cells stop cycling when they enter this phase

7. _____ includes G_1, S, G_2, and M

8. _____ undifferentiated or unspecialized cell

9. _____ replication of DNA occurs during this phase of the cell cycle

10. _____ type of cell division that occurs in sex cells

11. _____ a drug is labeled cell–cycle, M–phase specific; it affects this phase of the cell cycle

PART II: PUTTING IT ALL TOGETHER

MULTIPLE CHOICE

Directions. Choose the correct answer.

1. Which of the following is least characteristic of facilitated diffusion?

   a. passive transport
   b. "helper" molecule
   c. solute diffuses down its concentration gradient
   d. pumps solute from an area of low concentration to an area of high concentration

2. What is the process that uses energy to move a solute from an area of lower concentration to an area of higher concentration?

   a. diffusion
   b. facilitated diffusion
   c. osmosis
   d. active transport pump

Student Name _____

3. A hot dog bursts when it is boiled in water because the water

   a. is hypotonic.
   b. has too much salt.
   c. is hypertonic.
   d. is isotonic.

4. Perfume the skunk does "his thing." Which of the following words best indicates why you quickly become aware of Perfume's presence?

   a. diffusion
   b. Na$^+$/K$^+$ ATP pump
   c. active transport
   d. osmosis

5. Differentiation is

   a. a type of cell division.
   b. the process that refers to the specialization of cells.
   c. a type of passive transport.
   d. a form of active transport.

6. Which of the following best describes the cell membrane?

   a. nonselective
   b. selectively permeable
   c. impermeable
   d. exclusively lipid-soluble

7. Ribosomes are

   a. only found attached to the endoplasmic reticulum.
   b. located within the nucleus.
   c. concerned with protein synthesis.
   d. the power plants of the cell.

8. Which of the following terms is most related to the mitochondrion?

   a. mucus-secreting
   b. mRNA, tRNA
   c. protein synthesis
   d. energy-producing

9. Which of the following is most related to lysosomes?

   a. protein synthesis
   b. DNA
   c. bound and free
   d. "house cleaning"

10. Prophase, metaphase, anaphase, and telophase

    a. are stages of mitosis.
    b. are the resting phases of the cell cycle.
    c. occur during G_0 of the cell cycle.
    d. are transport mechanisms.

11. Interphase and mitosis

    a. refer to the resting phase of the cell cycle.
    b. are two phases of the cell cycle.
    c. do not include prophase, metaphase, anaphase, or telophase.
    d. are characteristic only of stem cells.

12. G_1, S, and G_2

    a. are stages of mitosis.
    b. occurs during interphase.
    c. occur only in stem cells.
    d. occur only in cancerous cells.

13. What is the underlying cause of the cellular effects of aging?

    a. increased numbers of organelles
    b. damage to DNA
    c. increased rate of cellular mitosis
    d. cellular shrinking

CASE STUDY

While performing breast self-examination, J.S. discovered a lump in the right upper quadrant of her left breast. She immediately contacted her physician and a biopsy was scheduled. The pathology report indicated a benign neoplasm composed of well-differentiated cells.

1. Which of the following is most characteristic of a benign neoplasm?

   a. metastatic
   b. well-differentiated cells
   c. malignant
   d. crablike

2. Which of the following words refers to the lump?

   a. biopsy
   b. metastasis
   c. Pap smear
   d. neoplasm

PART III: CHALLENGE YOURSELF!

GROUPS AND PUZZLE

1. Which group is incorrect?

   a. passive transport mechanisms: osmosis, diffusion, Na^+/K^+ ATP pump
   b. organelles: mitochondria, lysosomes, ribosomes
   c. transport mechanisms: diffusion, osmosis, filtration
   d. stages of mitosis: prophase, anaphase, metaphase, telophase

2. Which group is incorrect?

   a. organelles: mitochondria, lysosomes, ribosomes
   b. types of ribosomes: free, bound
   c. concentrations: isotonic, hypertonic, hypotonic
   d. active transport mechanisms: facilitated diffusion, osmosis, pinocytosis

3. Which group is incorrect?

   a. types of endoplasmic reticulum: rough and smooth
   b. types of endocytosis: pinocytosis, osmosis
   c. organelles: centrioles, microtubules, Golgi apparatus
   d. passive transport mechanisms: diffusion, osmosis, facilitated diffusion

PUZZLE

Hint: How to Get a Cell Mate

Directions. Perform the following functions on the Sequence of Words below. When all the functions have been performed, you are left with word(s) that are related to the hint. Record your answer below.

Functions: remove the following

1. control center of the cell

2. hair-like structures (2) on the surface of the cell membrane

3. passive transport mechanisms (4)

4. types of endoplasmic reticulum (2)

5. "power plants" of the cell

6. organelle that puts the finishing touches on a protein and then packages the protein for export

7. cellular eating and cellular drinking

8. phases of mitosis (4)

9. process of cellular specialization

Sequence of Words

ROUGHMETAPHASEDIFFERENTIATIONOSMOSISCILIAGOLGIAPPARATUSANAPHASEPI
NOCYTOSISFLAGELLUMNUCLEUSMITOCHONDRIATELOPHASEMITOSISFACILITATE
DDIFFUSIONDIFFUSIONPHAGOCYTOSISPROPHASEFILTRATIONSMOOTH

Answer: _____

4

Cell Metabolism

Answer Key: Textbook page references are provided as a guide for answering these questions. A complete answer key was provided for your instructor.

Objectives

1. Define metabolism, anabolism, and catabolism.

2. Explain the use of carbohydrates, proteins, and fats in the body.

3. Differentiate between the anaerobic and aerobic metabolism of carbohydrates.

4. Describe the structure of a nucleotide.

5. Describe the roles of DNA and RNA in protein synthesis.

6. Describe protein synthesis.

PART I: MASTERING THE BASICS

MATCHING

Carbohydrates, Fats, and Proteins

Directions. Match the following terms to the most appropriate definition by writing the correct letter in the space provided. Some terms may be used more than once. See text pp. 48-55.

A. glucose   F. glycogen   J. monosaccharides

B. amino acids   G. urea   K. lipids

C. nonessential amino acids   H. nitrogen   L. organic

D. disaccharides   I. essential amino acids   M. fatty acids and glycerol

E. cellulose

1. _____ refers to carbon-containing substances

2. _____ a nitrogen-containing waste product

3. _____ building blocks of lipids

4. _____ nondigestible polysaccharide found in plants

5. _____ protein contains this in addition to carbon, oxygen, and hydrogen

6. _____ building blocks that are joined together by peptide bonds

7. _____ amino acids that cannot be synthesized by the body and must therefore be obtained through dietary intake

8. _____ monosaccharide that provides the primary source of energy for the cells

9. _____ building blocks of protein

10. _____ sucrose, maltose, and lactose; sometimes called *double sugars*

11. _____ glucose, fructose, and galactose

12. _____ glucose is stored as this polysaccharide; it is also called *animal starch*

13. _____ amino acids that can be synthesized by the body

14. _____ classification of triglycerides and steroids

Student Name _____

MATCHING

Metabolism of Carbohydrates, Proteins, and Fats

Directions. Match the following terms to the most appropriate definition by writing the correct let-ter in the space provided. Some terms may be used more than once. See text pp. 48-55.

A. glycolysis

B. catabolism

C. CO_2, water, energy (ATP)

D. anabolism

E. enzyme

F. Krebs cycle

G. peptide bond

H. lactic acid

I. ketone bodies

1. _____ chemical reactions that build larger, more complex substances

2. _____ the amine group of alanine joins with the acid part of valine to form this

3. _____ are produced by the rapid, incomplete breakdown of fatty acids

4. _____ chemical reactions that degrade larger, more complex substances into simpler substances

5. _____ series of reactions that anaerobically break down glucose to lactic acid

6. _____ series of aerobic reactions that occur in the mitochondria

7. _____ in the absence of oxygen, pyruvic acid is converted to this substance

8. _____ end-products of the aerobic catabolism of glucose

9. _____ almost every chemical reaction in the body is catalyzed by this

10. _____ this series of anaerobic reactions occurs within the cytoplasm

MATCHING

Nucleotides: DNA and RNA

Directions. Match the following terms to the most appropriate definition by writing the correct letter in the space provided. Some terms may be used more than once. See text pp. 55-59.

A. DNA   C. deoxyribose   E. mRNA

B. tRNA   D. ribose   F. nucleotide

1. _____ double-stranded nucleic acid that contains the genetic code; called the *double helix*

2. _____ substance composed of phosphate, a sugar, and a base

3. _____ sugar found in RNA

4. _____ sugar found in DNA

5. _____ nucleotide that copies the genetic code from DNA in the nucleus

6. _____ nucleotide that carries individual amino acids from the cytoplasm to the ribosomes for assembly along the mRNA

7. _____ DNA and this nucleotide are involved in transcription

8. _____ mRNA and this nucleotide are involved in translation

9. _____ nucleotide that is confined to the nucleus

10. _____ nucleotide that does not use uracil in its coding; uses thymine instead

READ THE DIAGRAM

Directions. Refer to Figure 4-3 in the textbook and indicate if the following statements refer to column A or column B. Write A or B in the blanks below. See text p. 51.

1. _____ describes the anaerobic breakdown of glucose to lactic acid

2. _____ some of the chemical reactions occur within the mitochondria

3. _____ describes the complete breakdown of glucose into carbon dioxide, water, and energy

4. _____ most of the energy is formed in this pathway

5. _____ pyruvic acid enters the Krebs cycle for further catabolism

6. _____ all chemical reactions occur within the cytoplasm

7. _____ illustrates the role of the citric acid cycle in the catabolism of glucose

8. _____ includes oxygen-requiring reactions

9. _____ pyruvic acid is not converted to lactic acid

10. _____ chemical reactions that catabolize glucose incompletely

Student Name _____

PART II: PUTTING IT ALL TOGETHER

MULTIPLE CHOICE

Directions. Choose the correct answer.

1. Glucose

    a. is usually burned as fuel to get energy.
    b. can be converted to protein.
    c. can be converted to fat.
    d. must be converted to urea to be excreted from the body.

2. Urea

    a. is produced by the kidneys and eliminated in the bile.
    b. is a disaccharide.
    c. is a protein.
    d. is a nitrogen-containing substance produced in the liver and excreted in the urine.

3. Cellulose

    a. is animal starch.
    b. is the storage form of glucose.
    c. is a nitrogen-containing substance produced in the liver and excreted in the urine.
    d. is a nondigestible carbohydrate.

4. Which of the following best describes the composition of hormones, hemoglobin, and gamma globulins?

    a. carbohydrates
    b. proteins
    c. lipids
    d. glycerol

5. Gluconeogenesis is the process whereby

    a. glucose is converted to protein.
    b. fatty acids are combined with glycerol to form a monosaccharide.
    c. protein is used to make glucose.
    d. glucose is broken down to lactic acid.

6. Which of the following is required by the chemical reactions that occur within the mitochondria?

    a. lactic acid
    b. carbon dioxide
    c. oxygen
    d. cellulose

7. Glycogen

    a. combines with three fatty acids to make fat.
    b. is stored in the liver and skeletal muscle.
    c. is synthesized only in the pancreas.
    d. is a monosaccharide.

8. Why are you, unlike termites, unable to eat your wood house?

    a. Your teeth are not strong enough to chew wood.
    b. Your digestive tract would be injured by the wood splinters.
    c. You don't have the enzymes to digest the cellulose.
    d. The taste of wood is unappealing.

9. When blood sugar decreases, the glycogen in the liver is converted into which substance?

    a. protein
    b. ATP
    c. glucose
    d. lactic acid

10. Glycolysis

    a. is aerobic.
    b. forms CO_2 + water + energy.
    c. occurs only within the mitochondria.
    d. is anaerobic and cytoplasmic.

11. Which of the following is most related to the reactions of the Krebs cycle?

    a. anaerobic
    b. mitochondrial
    c. lactic acidosis
    d. urea-forming

12. Which of the following conditions is caused by a lack of oxygen in a critically ill patient?

    a. lactic acidosis
    b. cancer
    c. decreased blood glucose
    d. hypertension

13. Which of the following is least descriptive of ammonia?

    a. toxic to the brain
    b. accumulates in the presence of liver failure
    c. nitrogen-containing
    d. primary fuel for "running" the body

14. This protein substance acts as a catalyst, increasing the rate of a chemical reaction.

    a. urea
    b. enzyme
    c. mRNA
    d. ribose

15. If the bases of one side of DNA read: A-G-C-T, the complementary (opposite) DNA strand reads

    a. A-C-G-T.
    b. A-G-A-T.
    c. U-C-G-A.
    d. T-C-G-A.

16. Which of the following is most related to the storage of the genetic code?

    a. Krebs cycle
    b. glycolysis
    c. mitosis
    d. base-sequencing within the DNA molecule

17. With regard to base-pairing, thymine can only pair with which base?

    a. adenine
    b. uracil
    c. cytosine
    d. guanine

18. The bases in a strand of DNA read: T-C-C-A. The transcribed strand of mRNA reads

    a. A-G-G-T.
    b. G-C-G-A.
    c. U-C-C-T.
    d. A-G-G-U.

19. As a person ages, the body is less able to metabolize glucose efficiently, which results in elevated

    a. blood calcium levels.
    b. blood pressure.
    c. serum cholesterol levels.
    d. blood sugar levels.

20. Sue Crose is most related to

    a. Al Kalosis.
    b. Poly Saccharide.
    c. Di Saccharide.
    d. Cy T. O'Sine.

CASE STUDY

Until recently, 6-year-old Billie had no apparent health problems. About 1 week ago, she started to lose weight despite a healthy appetite. She urinated frequently and complained of being tired. Her mom noticed that she was very thirsty and was getting up in the middle of the night to urinate. On examination, her blood sugar was elevated and she had sugar and acetone in her urine. She was diagnosed with type 1 (juvenile-onset) diabetes mellitus.

1. Since the diabetic cells cannot utilize glucose, it accumulates in the blood, causing this condition.

    a. hypotension
    b. hyperglycemia
    c. lactic acidosis
    d. alkalosis

2. Because the diabetic person cannot use glucose, Billie metabolizes fatty acids rapidly and incompletely, thereby producing excessive amounts of this substance.

    a. enzymes
    b. ketone bodies
    c. glycogen
    d. urea

Student Name _____

3. Which of the following describes the effect of excess ketone bodies in the blood of a diabetic person?

    a. dehydration
    b. acidosis
    c. elevated blood pH
    d. hyperglycemia

PART III: CHALLENGE YOURSELF!

GROUPS AND PUZZLE

1. Which group is incorrect?

    a. monosaccharides: glucose, fructose, galactose
    b. nucleotides: DNA, RNA
    c. lipid-related structures: cholesterol, steroid, fatty acids
    d. amino acids: sucrose, maltose, lactose

2. Which group is incorrect?

    a. amino acids: essential, nonessential
    b. monosaccharides: glucose, fructose, galactose
    c. fatty acids: glycerol, glycogen
    d. ketone bodies: ketoacids, acetone

PUZZLE

Hint: Needs Oxygen… Name and Address

Directions. Perform the following functions on the Sequence of Words below. When all the functions have been performed, you are left with word(s) that are related to the hint. Record your answer below.

Functions: remove the following

1.   building blocks of proteins

2.   monosaccharides

3.   nitrogen-containing waste product

4.   series of reactions that degrade glucose to lactic acid; anaerobic and cytoplasmic

5.   series of reactions that makes glucose from protein breakdown products

6.   disaccharides

7.   building blocks of fats

8.   storage form of glucose

9.   term that includes anabolism and catabolism

10.   nucleotide that stores the genetic code within the nucleus

11.   nucleotide that carries the genetic code from the nucleus to the ribosomes in the cytoplasm

12.   two sugars found within DNA and RNA

13.   four bases found in DNA

Sequence of Words

GUANINERIBOSEDNAGLUCONEOGENESISSUCROSEGLUCOSECYTOSINEMALTOSEG
ALACTOSEUREAFATTYACIDSGLYCOGENGLYCEROLMETABOLISMDEOXYRIBOSEAMI
NOACIDSTHYMINEHANSKREBSMITOCHONDRIONADENINEGLYCOLYSISFRUCTOSEL
ACTOSEmRNA

Answer: _____

5

Microbiology Basics

Answer Key: Textbook page references are provided as a guide for answering these questions. A complete answer key was provided for your instructor.

Objectives

1. Define disease and infection.

2. Describe the types of bacteria by shape and staining characteristics.

3. List the characteristics of the different types of pathogens.

4. Define portals of exit and portals of entry.

5. List common ways in which infections are spread.

6. Identify the microbiological principles described in Six Germ-Laden Stories.

PART I: MASTERING THE BASICS

MATCHING

Germs, Worms, and Terms

Directions. Match the following terms to the most appropriate definition by writing the correct letter in the space provided. See text pp. 63-68.

A. parasites

B. vector

C. normal flora

D. gram stain

E. zoonosis

F. nosocomial

G. disease

H. portals of entry

I. pathogen

J. infection

K. portals of exit

1. _____   failure of the body to function normally

2. _____   disease-causing organism

3. _____   disease caused by a pathogen or its toxin

4. _____   an object (living or nonliving) that transfers a pathogen from one organism to another

5. _____   organisms that normally and harmoniously live in or on the human body

6. _____   organisms that require a living host in which to survive

7. _____   routes by which pathogens enter the body

8. _____   hospital-acquired infection

9. _____   dye used to identify different kinds of bacteria

10. _____   an animal disease that is transmissible to humans

11. _____   routes by which pathogens leave the body

MATCHING

Pathogens

Directions. Match the following terms to the most appropriate definition by writing the correct letter in the space provided. Some terms may be used more than once. See text pp. 64-67.

A. bacteria   C. fungi   E. worms

B. virus   D. protozoa   F. arthropods

1. _____ coccus, bacillus, curved rod

2. _____ acts as a parasite to the infected cell

3. _____ mycotic infections

4. _____ plantlike organisms such as mushrooms

5. _____ single-cell, animal-like microbes

6. _____ chlamydia and rickettsia

7. _____ from the Latin meaning *poison*

8. _____ amebas, ciliates, flagellates, sporozoa

9. _____ diplococcus, streptococcus, staphylococcus

10. _____ consists of RNA or DNA surrounded by a protein shell

11. _____ yeasts and molds

12. _____ arrangement: pairs, chains, bunches of grapes

13. _____ vibrio, spirillum, spirochete

14. _____ helminths

15. _____ ectoparasites

16. _____ ascarides, trichinae, flukes

17. _____ animals with jointed legs, including insects and ticks

18. _____ Gram (+) and Gram (−)

MATCHING

Germer-Laden Stories

Directions. Match the following stories to the most appropriate description by writing the correct letter in the space provided. The stories may be used more than once. See text pp. 68-71.

A. Dr. Semmelweis Screams "Wash Those Mitts"

B. Flora and Her Vaginal Itch

C. Rick, Nick, and the Sick Tick

D. Why Typhoid Mary Needed to Lose Her Gallbladder

E. Pox News Alert

F. The Chief of Staph Reports

1. _____ focuses on handwashing, dirty hands, and nosocomial infection

2. _____ great example of the carrier state and disease transmission by the fecal-oral route

3. _____ focuses on microorganisms and superinfection

4. _____ Committee on Pimples and Boils

5. _____ Varicella-zoster

6. _____ salmonella hides in bile

7. _____ the injected saliva was teeming with rickettsia

8. _____ the conclusion of this tormented scientist: "Puerperal fever is caused by conveyance to the pregnant woman of 'putrid particles' derived from living organisms, through the agency of the examining finger"

9. _____ great example of zoonosis

10. _____ Gram (+) organism with many drug-resistant strains

11. _____ describes an insect as a "reservoir of infection"

12. _____ describes the overgrowth of *Candida albicans* (yeast), causing itching and discharge

13. _____ vesicular skin lesions

14. _____ MRSA, MRSA, MRSA

15. _____ describes the alteration of the normal flora by antibiotics

16. _____ this streptococcal infection began in the uterus and progressed to peritonitis, generalized septicemia, and death

17. _____ Aureus and his golden exudate

18. _____ illustrates disease transmission by an arthropod vector

19. _____ scalded skin syndrome, impetigo, and food poisoning

20. _____ childhood illness and shingles

21. _____ defines transovarian passage

22. _____ differentiates between a communicable and contagious disease

23. _____ Salmonella-laced dinner

Student Name _____

PART II: PUTTING IT ALL TOGETHER

MULTIPLE CHOICE

Directions. Choose the correct answer.

1. Ringworm
   a. refers to a heminthic infection.
   b. is a mycotic infection.
   c. is also called impetigo.
   d. is due to a strain of staphylococcus.

2. Person-to-person, environment-to-person, and tiny animal-to-person refers to the
   a. staining characteristics of pathogens.
   b. size of the pathogens.
   c. spread or transmission of the pathogens.
   d. sensitivity to chemotherapy.

3. Which of the following is a true statement about bacteria?
   a. All bacteria are pathogenic.
   b. The spread of bacterial infections requires arthropod vectors.
   c. Pathogenic bacteria cause mycotic infections.
   d. Most bacteria perform useful functions; fewer are pathogenic.

4. Mycotic infections are
   a. caused by Gram (–) bacilli.
   b. viral infections.
   c. fungal infections.
   d. always zoonotic.

5. Infection by *Candida albicans*
   a. is viral and therefore unresponsive to antibiotics.
   b. only occurs in the vagina.
   c. often appears as a superinfection following antibiotic therapy.
   d. requires a biological vector such as a tick.

6. Viruses
   a. are surrounded by a rigid cell wall.
   b. are sensitive to penicillin.
   c. are the smallest of the infectious agents and are fragments of either RNA or DNA surrounded by a protein shell.
   d. classified as Gram (+) and Gram (–).

7. Amebas, flagellates, ciliates, and sporozoa are
   a. anaerobic, spore-forming bacteria.
   b. protozoa.
   c. fungi.
   d. rickettsia.

8. An anthelmintic exerts its therapeutic effects against
   a. Gram (–) bacteria.
   b. all spore-forming microorganisms.
   c. viruses.
   d. worms.

9. A young child has pinworms. Which observation will usually be made by the parent?
   a. malaise, fever, and generalized wasting
   b. abdominal swelling and severe diarrhea
   c. nausea, vomiting, and weight loss
   d. perianal pruritus

10. These arthropods live on the surface of the body and cause itching and discomfort, but are not life-threatening.
    a. ectoparasites
    b. normal flora
    c. viruses
    d. protozoa

11. With regard to the spread of malaria, the mosquito is the
    a. causative organism of malaria.
    b. arthropod vector.
    c. fomite.
    d. pathogen.

12. Which of the following is least related to staphylococcus?
    a. Gram (+) bacterium
    b. impetigo, food poisoning, and scalded skin syndrome
    c. chickenpox and shingles
    d. usual cause of most skin infections

13. *Clostridium tetani*

    a. is an ectoparasite.
    b. grows best in a puncture wound under anaerobic conditions.
    c. is Gram (+) and aerobic.
    d. grows best on the skin surface.

14. Which of the following is not characteristic of *Candida albicans*?

    a. mycotic infection
    b. is a member of the normal flora of the mouth, digestive tract, and vagina
    c. is a spore-forming anaerobe like the clostridium microbes
    d. can cause a superinfection

15. A pox is

    a. usually responsive to an antibiotic cream.
    b. a mycotic infection.
    c. a vesicular skin lesion.
    d. a luetic lesion.

16. The Great pox, chancre, and luetic lesions are associated with

    a. gonorrhea.
    b. giardiasis.
    c. impetigo.
    d. syphilis.

PART III: CHALLENGE YOURSELF!

GROUPS AND PUZZLE

1. Which group is incorrect?

    a. arrangement of cocci: diplococcus, streptococcus, staphylococcus
    b. bacteria: coccus, bacillus, curved rod
    c. curved rods: vibrio, spirillum, fungus
    d. arthropod vectors: fleas, ticks, lice, mosquitoes

2. Which group is incorrect?

    a. bacteria: coccus, bacillus, curved rod
    b. arthropod vectors: fleas, ticks, lice, mosquitoes
    c. protozoa: amebas, ciliates, flagellates, sporozoa
    d. contagious diseases: measles, chickenpox, urinary bladder infection

3. Which group is incorrect?

    a. arrangement of cocci: diplococcus, streptococcus, bacillus
    b. arthropod vectors: fleas, ticks, lice, mosquitoes
    c. protozoa: amebas, ciliates, flagellates, sporozoa
    d. contagious diseases: measles, chickenpox, mumps

PUZZLE

Hint: Fun Guy or Fungi

Directions. Perform the following functions on the Sequence of Words below. When all the functions have been performed, you are left with word(s) that are related to the hint. Record your answer below.

Functions: remove the following

1. types of bacteria

2. hospital-acquired infection

3. disease-causing microorganism

4. organisms that normally and harmoniously live in or on the human body without causing disease

5. two types of cocci

6. organism that requires a living host

7. a parasitic worm

8. a tiny parasite that is composed primarily strands of DNA or RNA

9. refers to mites, lice, and ticks

10. an animal disease that is transmissible to humans

11. main types (4) of protozoa

Sequence of Words

AMEBASCOCCUSPARASITENOSOCOMIALCILIATESSTAPHECTOPARASITESFLAGEL
LATESZOONOSISNORMALFLORAVIRUSSPOROZOABACILLUSHELMINTHMOLDCURV
EDRODSSTREPPATHOGEN

Answer: _____

BODY TOON

Hint: Plugged in... "la...la...la"

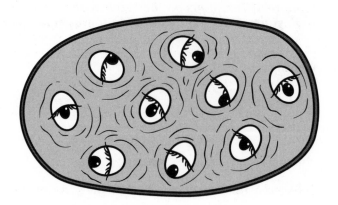

Tissues and Membranes

Answer Key: Textbook page references are provided as a guide for answering these questions. A complete answer key was provided for your instructor.

Objectives

1. List the four basic types of tissues.

2. Describe the functions of epithelial, connective, muscle, and nervous tissue.

3. Explain how epithelial tissue is classified.

4. Differentiate between endocrine and exocrine glands.

5. List the types of epithelial and connective tissue membranes.

6. Differentiate between mucous and serous membranes.

PART I: MASTERING THE BASICS

MATCHING

Types of Tissue

Directions. Match the following terms to the most appropriate definition by writing the correct letter in the space provided. Some terms may be used more than once. See text pp. 76-85.

A. epithelial tissue

B. connective tissue

C. muscle tissue

D. nervous tissue

1. _____ tissue that is avascular and is nourished from the underlying connective tissue

2. _____ osseous tissue

3. _____ attached to a basement membrane

4. _____ blood, bone, cartilage, and adipose tissue

5. _____ neurons and glia

6. _____ classified as squamous, cuboidal, and columnar

7. _____ classified as simple or stratified

8. _____ has the greatest amount of intercellular matrix of the four tissue types

9. _____ classified as skeletal, smooth, and cardiac

10. _____ type of tissue that forms ligaments that attach muscle to bone

11. _____ dense fibrous, reticular, and areolar

12. _____ a specialized type of this tissue stores fat

13. _____ a sarcoma arises from this type of tissue

14. _____ a carcinoma arises from this type of tissue

15. _____ primary functions include secretion, absorption, excretion, and protection

16. _____ most abundant of the four tissue types

17. _____ forms the epidermis

18. _____ endocrine and exocrine glands arise from this type of tissue

19. _____ binds together parts of the body; examples include ligaments, tendons, capsules, and fascia

20. _____ has two surfaces; one surface is always unattached or free, such as the surface of the outer skin and the lining of the mouth

21. _____ chondrocytes and oseocytes

22. _____ transitional; found in stretchy organs like the urinary bladder

Student Name _____

MATCHING

Membranes

Directions. Match the following terms to the most appropriate definition by writing the correct letter in the space provided. See text pp. 85-87.

A. visceral pleura

B. synovial membrane

C. visceral peritoneum

D. parietal pleura

E. pericardium

F. parietal peritoneum

G. cutaneous membrane

H. mucous membrane

I. connective tissue membrane

1. _____ membrane lining all body cavities that opens to the outside of the body

2. _____ connective tissue membrane that lines the cavities of joints

3. _____ skin

4. _____ serous membrane that covers the outside of each lung

5. _____ serous membrane that lines the inner wall of the abdominopelvic cavity

6. _____ serous membrane that lines the organs of the abdominopelvic cavity

7. _____ serous membrane that lines the walls of the thoracic cavity

8. _____ synovial membrane and periosteum

9. _____ lines the mouth, nose, and respiratory passages

10. _____ sling that supports the heart

READ THE DIAGRAM

Directions. Referring to the illustration, write the numbers on the lines provided below. See text p. 86.

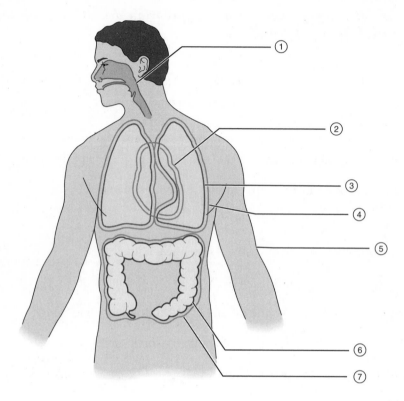

1. _____ an example of a mucous membrane

2. _____ cutaneous membrane

3. _____ parietal peritoneum

4. _____ the serous membrane that "hugs" the outer side of the lung

5. _____ a pericardial membrane

6. _____ visceral peritoneum

7. _____ serous membrane that "hugs" the inner walls of the thoracic cavity

COLOR AND DRAW

Directions. Using the diagram above, color the following structures.

1. Color the parietal pleura *blue*.
2. Color the visceral pleura *green*.
3. Color the intrapleural space *yellow*.
4. Draw the diaphragm.

Student Name _____

PART II: PUTTING IT ALL TOGETHER

MULTIPLE CHOICE

Directions. Choose the correct answer.

1. The parietal and visceral pleura

    a. are mucous membranes.
    b. secrete small amounts of serous fluid.
    c. are located in the abdominal cavity.
    d. surround the heart.

2. Epithelial tissue

    a. has extensive intercellular material.
    b. forms large continuous sheets of tissue.
    c. forms tendons, ligaments, and capsules.
    d. is described as visceral and parietal.

3. Glandular tissue

    a. is found only within the abdominal organs.
    b. arises from epithelial tissue.
    c. is classified as dense fibrous and areolar.
    d. stores fat.

4. Mucous membrane

    a. forms the pleurae.
    b. forms the peritoneal membranes.
    c. lines the respiratory tract.
    d. is a type of connective tissue membrane.

5. Squamous, cuboidal, and columnar

    a. refer to the layers of epithelial tissue.
    b. are types of nervous tissue.
    c. are shapes of epithelial tissue.
    d. are found only within the thoracic cavity.

6. Simple and stratified

    a. refer to the layers of epithelial tissue.
    b. are types of nervous tissue.
    c. are shapes of epithelial tissue.
    d. are found only within the thoracic cavity.

7. Which of the following membranes is confined to the thoracic cavity?

    a. meninges
    b. peritoneum
    c. synovial membranes
    d. pleurae

8. Because this type of tissue is so thin, it is concerned primarily with the movement of various substances across the membranes from one body compartment to another.

    a. connective tissue
    b. neuroglia
    c. simple squamous epithelium
    d. cartilage

9. Which of the following is most related to glandular epithelium?

    a. simple cuboidal epithelium
    b. skeletal, cardiac, and smooth
    c. tendons, ligaments
    d. adipose

10. Which of the following is related to endocrine glands?

    a. pleura and peritoneum
    b. serous and mucous
    c. ductless glands
    d. visceral and parietal

11. In which type of tissue is the intercellular matrix hardest?

    a. blood
    b. bone
    c. simple squamous epithelium
    d. adipose

12. Which of the following is most descriptive of cartilage?

    a. squamous cell epithelium
    b. basement membrane
    c. hyaline and elastic
    d. endocrine and exocrine

13. Which of the following does not appear in the thoracic cavity?

    a. serous membranes
    b. pleural membranes
    c. serous fluid
    d. peritoneal membrane

14. Which of the following best describes scar tissue?

    a. sarcoma
    b. regeneration
    c. meninges
    d. fibrosis

15. Which of the following are described as parietal and visceral?

    a. mucous membranes
    b. serous membranes
    c. synovial membranes
    d. meninges

16. This condition is due to prolonged pressure that causes a decrease in the blood supply to the tissues.

    a. peritonitis
    b. lactic acidosis
    c. decubitus ulcer
    d. meningitis

17. Which word is most descriptive of gangrenous tissue?

    a. necrotic
    b. scar
    c. fibrotic
    d. malignant

18. Why do tissues become stiffer and less efficient with aging?

    a. The epithelial membranes become thicker.
    b. There is an increase in intracellular fluid.
    c. There is a decrease in collagen and elastin in connective tissue.
    d. Muscle and nerve tissue hypertrophy.

19. This person "has heart."

    a. Perry T. O'Neum
    b. Addie Pose
    c. Perry Cardium
    d. Hy A. Lin

CASE STUDY

Six-year-old J.P. complained to her mom that she had a pain in her stomach. Her mom attributed the pain to too much junk food and suggested that she go to bed early. At 4 AM, J.P. awoke with severe abdominal pain, a high fever, and a rigid and boardlike abdomen. Her physician admitted her to the hospital with a diagnosis of a ruptured appendix.

1. Which of the following is likely to develop in response to the ruptured appendix as waste—feces—leaks into the abdominopelvic cavity?

    a. peritonitis
    b. pleurisy
    c. hemorrhoids
    d. pericarditis

2. Which of the following became inflamed?

    a. pleura
    b. serous membrane
    c. meninges
    d. synovial membrane

Student Name _____

PART III: CHALLENGE YOURSELF

GROUPS AND PUZZLE

1. Which group is incorrect?

   a. appearance of epithelial tissue: squamous, cuboidal, columnar
   b. types of muscle: skeletal, cardiac, and adipose
   c. types of nervous tissue: neurons and neuroglia
   d. types of fibers: collagen, elastin, and reticular

2. Which group is incorrect?

   a. shapes of epithelial tissue: squamous, cuboidal, and columnar
   b. types of connective tissue: adipose, areolar, dense fibrous
   c. layers of epithelial tissue: simple and stratified
   d. serous membranes in thoracic cavity: pleura, pericardium, peritoneum

3. Which group is incorrect?

   a. layers of connective tissue: simple and stratified
   b. types of tissues: epithelial, connective, nerve, and muscle
   c. types of nervous tissue: neurons and neuroglia
   d. types of connective tissue: areola, dense fibrous, reticular, cartilage, bone, and blood

PUZZLE

Hint: Scales, Columns, and Cubes

Directions. Perform the following functions on the Sequence of Words below. When all the functions have been performed, you are left with word(s) that are related to the hint. Record your answer below.

Functions: remove the following

1. examples of connective tissue (6)

2. two types of nervous tissue

3. types of muscle tissue (3)

4. two types of glands formed from glandular epithelium

5. three serous membranes

6. types of connective tissue that have a watery intercellular matrix

7. type of membrane that lines the digestive and respiratory tracts

8. connective tissue membrane that covers bone

9. connective tissue membrane that covers the brain and the spinal cord

Sequence of Words

MENINGESCARTILAGEEXOCRINESMOOTHPERITONEUMTENDONSNEUROGLIAARE
OLARSKELETALPERIOSTEUMBONEPERICARDIUMENDOCRINEBLOODEPITHELIA
LTISSUEADIPOSELYMPHPLEURALIGAMENTSCARDIACMUCOUSNEURON

Answer: _____

Integumentary System and Body Temperature

Answer Key: Textbook page references are provided as a guide for answering these questions. A complete answer key was provided for your instructor.

Objectives

1. Describe the two layers of skin: epidermis and dermis.

2. Define stratum germinativum and stratum corneum.

3. List the two major functions of the subcutaneous layer.

4. List the factors that influence the color of the skin.

5. Describe the accessory structures of the skin: hair, nails, and glands.

6. List six functions of the skin.

7. Describe how the skin helps to regulate temperature.

8. Explain four processes by which the body loses heat.

PART I: MASTERING THE BASICS

MATCHING

The Skin

Directions. Match the following terms to the most appropriate definition by writing the correct letter in the space provided. Some terms may be used more than once. See text pp. 91-93.

A. dermis
B. subcutaneous layer
C. epidermis

D. keratin
E. stratum germinativum
F. stratum corneum

G. integument
H. dermatology

1. _____   the study of the skin and skin disorders

2. _____   contains the stratum germinativum and the stratum corneum

3. _____   contains adipose tissue

4. _____   layer of skin that contains the blood vessels, nerves, and sensory receptors

5. _____   epidermal layer that forms the bathtub ring

6. _____   layer underneath the epidermis

7. _____   layer of epidermis that continuously produces millions of cells every day

8. _____   a protein in the skin that flattens, hardens, and makes the skin water-resistant

9. _____   surface layer of the epidermis that makes up most of the epidermal thickness

10. _____   layer that insulates the body from extreme temperature changes and anchors the skin to the underlying structures

11. _____   hypodermis

12. _____   another name for the skin

13. _____   desquamation and exfoliation refer to this epidermal layer

14. _____   another name for the cutaneous membrane

15. _____   this epidermal layer forms corns and calluses

Student Name _____

MATCHING

Glands of the Skin

Directions. Match the following terms to the most appropriate definition by writing the correct letter in the space provided. Some terms may be used more than once. See text pp. 96-98.

A. ceruminous   C. eccrine   E. mammary

B. apocrine   D. sebaceous

1. _____ oil glands

2. _____ a blackhead is formed when this gland becomes blocked by accumulated oil and debris

3. _____ a pimple is formed when the sebum of this blocked gland becomes infected

4. _____ sweat glands that cause body odor and are responsible for sex attractants in animals

5. _____ babies are born with a "cream cheese-like" covering called *vernix caseosa* that is secreted by these glands

6. _____ these glands and the apocrine glands are classified as sudoriferous glands

7. _____ sweat glands that are usually associated with hair follicles and are found in the axillary and genital areas

8. _____ sweat glands that respond to emotional stress and also become activated when a person is sexually aroused

9. _____ sweat glands that play the most important role in temperature regulation

10. _____ milk-secreting glands that are classified as modified sweat glands

11. _____ modified sweat glands that secrete earwax

MATCHING

Skin Characteristics and Conditions

Directions. Match the following terms to the most appropriate definition by writing the correct letter in the space provided. See text pp. 94-96.

A. jaundice   E. melanin   I. alopecia

B. freckles   F. albinism   J. flushing

C. melanoma   G. carotene   K. pallor

D. cyanosis   H. vitiligo

1. _____ pigment that darkens the skin; the pigment-secreting cells are stimulated by ultraviolet radiation (e.g., "tanning")

2. _____ condition in which no melanin is secreted

3. _____ loss of pigment in the skin that creates patches of white skin

4. _____ melanin is concentrated in local areas; benign

5. _____ highly malignant form of skin cancer that arises from melanocytes

6. _____ substance that gives persons of Asian descent a slight yellowish skin coloring

7. _____ caused by vasodilation of the dermal blood vessels

8. _____ caused by vasoconstriction of the dermal blood vessels

9. _____ condition in which the skin has a bluish tint caused by a diminished amount of oxygen in the blood

10. _____ color change caused by hypoxemia

11. _____ hair loss

12. _____ yellowing of the skin caused by an accumulation of bilirubin in the skin

13. _____ described as *ashen*

Student Name _____

MATCHING

Skin: Water and Temperature

Directions. Match the following terms to the most appropriate definition by writing the correct letter in the space provided. See text pp. 98-100.

A. sensible perspiration   D. thermoregulation   G. core temperature

B. hypothalamus   E. shivering thermogenesis H. shell temperature

C. insensible perspiration   F. modes of heat loss   I. nonshivering thermogenesis

1. _____ temperature within the cranial, thoracic, and abdominal cavities

2. _____ mechanisms whereby the body balances heat production and heat loss

3. _____ about 500 mL/day of water is lost through the skin

4. _____ eccrine glands are responsible for this type of perspiration

5. _____ heat production due to continuous contractions of skeletal muscles when cold

6. _____ evaporation, conduction, convection, and radiation

7. _____ heat production caused by the metabolism of brown fat in the neonate

8. _____ temperature of the surface areas such as the skin, mouth, and axilla

9. _____ thermostat of the body

PART II: PUTTING IT ALL TOGETHER

MULTIPLE CHOICE

Directions. Choose the correct answer.

1. Which of the following is least true of the epidermis?
    a. thin outer layer of the skin
    b. contains a rich supply of blood vessels
    c. contains the stratum germinativum and stratum corneum
    d. cells become keratinized

2. Epidermal cells become keratinized meaning that they
    a. appear yellow.
    b. are hardened and water-resistant.
    c. have been replaced by connective tissue.
    d. appear cyanotic.

3. The dermis

    a. contains the stratum germinativum and the stratum corneum.
    b. contains the blood vessels that oxygenate the epidermis.
    c. cannot stretch.
    d. is the target for subcutaneous injections.

4. The subcutaneous layer

    a. is located directly under the epidermis.
    b. contains the stratum germinativum.
    c. is the layer that tans when exposed to ultraviolet radiation.
    d. supports the dermis.

5. Why do we feel the heat intensely on a hot and humid day?

    a. Heat loss increases because of an increase in evaporation.
    b. Vasoconstriction traps heat in the body.
    c. Heat loss decreases because of a decrease in evaporation.
    d. The arrector pili muscles work overtime.

6. Epidermal cells desquamate or exfoliate, meaning that they

    a. become yellow.
    b. form calluses.
    c. slough.
    d. synthesize vitamin D in response to ultraviolet radiation.

7. Which of the following is true of the stratum germinativum?

    a. the cells are dead and are constantly sloughed
    b. is part of the dermis
    c. originates in the hypodermis
    d. replenishes the cells of the epidermis that have sloughed

8. The skin over your knuckles is wrinkled and creased because it is

    a. keratinized.
    b. avascular.
    c. dead.
    d. anchored directly to bone.

9. Albinism, freckles, vitiligo, moles, and tanning are conditions that are all associated with which of the following?

    a. cancer
    b. melanin
    c. cell necrosis
    d. keratinization

10. Alopecia is most likely to occur in a

    a. tanned patient.
    b. cyanotic patient.
    c. patient who is being treated with anticancer drugs.
    d. patient with vitiligo.

11. Which of the following is related to eccrine glands?

    a. classified as endocrine glands
    b. secrete sebum
    c. secrete sweat
    d. are called *oil glands*

12. Nonshivering thermogenesis in the neonate

    a. is accomplished by contracting skeletal muscles.
    b. is due to the contraction of the arrector pili muscles.
    c. is a heat-loss mechanism.
    d. is accomplished by the metabolism of brown fat.

13. Which of the following people is most likely to exhibit hirsutism?

    a. person who is chronically hypoxic (low oxygen) because of a lung disease
    b. a person who has liver failure and therefore has excess bilirubin in his blood
    c. a woman who is taking testosterone
    d. a male who has been castrated (loss of testicular function)

14. Which of the following people is most likely to exhibit clubbing?

    a. person who is chronically hypoxic (low oxygen) because of a lung disease
    b. a person who has liver failure and therefore has excess bilirubin in his blood
    c. a woman who is taking testosterone
    d. a male who has been castrated (loss of testicular function)

15. Which patient is most likely to require an escharotomy?

    a. a person who is cyanotic
    b. a person with severe digital clubbing
    c. a severely burned patient
    d. a person with drug-induced urticaria

16. Why does the skin become dry, coarse, and itchy in the older person? There is

    a. a decrease in the amount of adipose tissue.
    b. an increase in the blood flow to the skin.
    c. an increased fragility of the skin.
    d. decreased sebaceous gland activity in the skin.

17. Why do older people tend to feel cold?

    a. There is a decrease in the amount of adipose tissue under the skin.
    b. There is an increase of blood flow to the skin, resulting in excess cooling.
    c. Metabolic rate increases with age.
    d. Keratinization decreases with age.

18. Whose skin is the lightest?

    a. Mel A. Nin
    b. Al Bino
    c. Cy A. Nosis
    d. Mel A. Noma

19. This guy is a flake.

    a. Al Bino
    b. Cy Anosis
    c. Dan Druff
    d. Mel A. N. O'Cyte

CASE STUDY

Sixteen-year-old Kevin was involved in a car accident and suffered full-thickness burns over both lower extremities. Upon admission to the hospital, he was given large amounts of fluid intravenously and placed on sterile sheets.

1. What information can be obtained from the Rule of Nines? Kevin

    a. suffered full-thickness burns.
    b. was burned over 36% of his body.
    c. should be experiencing excruciating pain.
    d. was burned over 75% of his body.

2. What is the primary reason that Kevin requires large amounts of intravenous fluids?

    a. He has not had anything to drink since the accident.
    b. The loss of skin causes the loss of large volumes of body fluid.
    c. Sterile sheets pull water out of the burn site.
    d. He is thirsty.

3. Despite his severe burns, Kevin might not require heavy doses of pain medicine because

    a. he is immobile and not moving the injured site.
    b. the burn site has not yet become infected.
    c. the pain receptors in the dermis have been destroyed.
    d. the melanin within the skin acts as a pain reliever.

PART III: CHALLENGE YOURSELF!

GROUPS AND PUZZLE

1. Which of the following is incorrect?

    a. melanin concentrations: albinism, freckles, moles, vitiligo
    b. major exocrine glands of the skin: sebaceous glands and sweat glands
    c. types of sweat glands: eccrine and sebaceous
    d. modes of heat loss: conduction, convection, evaporation, radiation

2. Which of the following is incorrect?

    a. modes of heat loss: conduction, convection, evaporation, radiation
    b. layers of the skin: epidermis and dermis
    c. layers of the epidermis: subcutaneous, stratum germinativum
    d. major exocrine glands of the skin: sebaceous glands and sweat glands

3. Which of the following is incorrect?

    a. layers of the skin: epidermis and dermis
    b. skin color changes: cyanosis, jaundice, and tanning
    c. modes of heat loss: conduction, convection, evaporation, radiation
    d. layers of the dermis: stratum corneum and stratum germinativum

PUZZLE

Hint: Red, White, and Blue of Skin

Directions. Perform the following functions on the Sequence of Words below. When all the functions have been performed, you are left with word(s) that are related to the hint. Record your answer below.

Functions: remove the following

1. The two types of sudoriferous glands
2. The two layers of skin
3. Two layers epithelium
4. Cells that secrete a dark "tanning" pigment in response to exposure to UV radiation
5. The layer upon which the dermis sits
6. The cream cheese-like substance that covers the skin of the newborn infant
7. The pigment that causes jaundice
8. The condition that is caused by a lack of melanin
9. The protein that makes the skin water-resistant
10. Glands most associated with the blackhead

Sequence of Words

SUBCUTANEOUSEPIDERMISSTRATUMCORNEUMERYTHEMAECCRINESEBACEOUSAPO
CRINEDERMISSTRATUMGERMINATIVUMPALLORVERNIXCASEOSAMELANOCYTESBILI
RUBINCYANOSISKERATINALBINISM

Answer: _____, _____, _____

8

Skeletal System

Answer Key: Textbook page references are provided as a guide for answering these questions. A complete answer key was provided for your instructor.

Objectives

1. List the functions of the skeletal system.

2. Describe the structure of a long bone.

3. Describe the roles of osteoblasts and osteoclasts.

4. List the bones of the axial skeleton.

5. List the bones of the appendicular skeleton.

6. Label important landmarks for selected bones on the skeleton.

7. List the main types and functions of joints.

8. Describe the types of joint movement.

PART I: MASTERING THE BASICS

MATCHING

Long Bone

Directions. Match the following terms to the most appropriate definition by writing the correct letter in the space provided. See text pp. 107-111.

A. osteocyte

B. osteoblast

C. bone marrow

D. compact bone

E. spongy bone

F. haversian system

G. trabeculae

H. diaphysis

I. epiphyseal disc

J. endosteum

K. osteoclast

L. medullary cavity

M. periosteum

N. epiphysis

O. articular cartilage

1. _____ dense, hard type of bone

2. _____ bony plates found in spongy bone

3. _____ band of hyaline cartilage at ends of long bone; longitudinal bone growth occurs here

4. _____ tough outer connective tissue covering the diaphysis of a long bone

5. _____ hollow center of the shaft of the bone

6. _____ found on the outer surface of the epiphysis

7. _____ microscopic unit of compact bone; also called an *osteon*

8. _____ mature bone cell

9. _____ inner lining of the medullary cavity of a long bone

10. _____ the shaft of a long bone

11. _____ site of blood cell formation

12. _____ eroding activity of this cell remodels and expands the medullary cavity

13. _____ a bone-building cell

14. _____ cancellous bone

15. _____ the enlarged end of a long bone

16. _____ this type of bone has a punched or "Swiss cheese" appearance

17. _____ called the *growth plate*

18. _____ this cell is responsible for bone resorption

Student Name _____

MATCHING

Skull

Directions. Match the following terms to the most appropriate definition by writing the correct letter in the space provided. Some terms may be used more than once. See text pp. 114-118.

A. maxilla
B. mandible
C. palatine bones
D. frontal

E. parietal
F. external auditory meatus
G. occipital
H. sphenoid

I. zygomatic bones
J. temporal
K. ethmoid
L. fontanels

1. __B__ lower jaw bone; contains the lower teeth

2. _____ opening in the temporal bone for the ear

3. _____ upper jaw bone; contains the upper teeth

4. _____ cheekbones; also form part of the orbits of the eyes

5. _____ forms the top and sides of the skull

6. _____ forms the bony structure of the nasal cavity

7. _____ forms the chin

8. _____ forms the floor and back wall of the cranium

9. _____ the large hole in this bone is called the *foramen magnum*

10. _____ forms the posterior part of the hard palate and the floor of the nasal cavity

11. _____ butterfly-shaped bone that forms part of the floor and sides of the cranium; the sella turcica houses the pituitary gland

12. _____ forms the forehead

13. __L__ means "little fountain," the baby's soft spots

14. _____ on the sides of the head close to the ears

15. _____ contains the external auditory meatus, styloid process, zygomatic process, and mastoid process

16. _____ articulates with the temporal bone to form a freely movable joint

17. _____ the condyles of this bone sit on the atlas

18. _____ the M in TMJ

19. _____ the T in TMJ

20. _____ bone that articulates with the parietal bone at the coronal suture

READ THE DIAGRAM

The Skull

Directions. Referring to the diagram, write the numbers in the blanks below. See text p. 115.

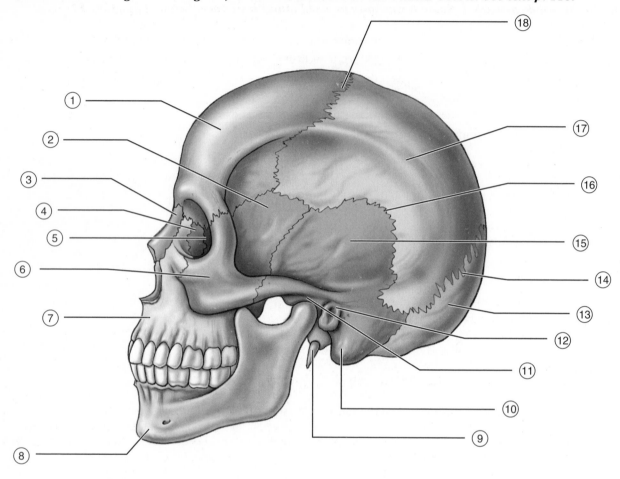

1. _____ mandible
2. _____ external auditory meatus
3. _____ maxilla
4. _____ zygomatic bone
5. _____ parietal bone
6. _____ styloid process
7. _____ mastoid process
8. _____ frontal bone
9. _____ bone that contains the foramen magnum
10. _____ bone that contains the external auditory meatus, styloid process, zygomatic process, and mastoid process
11. _____ bone that articulates with the temporal bone to form a freely movable joint
12. _____ the immovable joint between the frontal and parietal bones

Student Name _____

MATCHING

Thoracic Cage

Directions. Match the following terms to the most appropriate definition by writing the correct letter in the space provided. Some terms may be used more than once. See text pp. 120-121.

A. false ribs	D. manubrium	G. costal angle
B. true ribs	E. xiphoid process	H. manubriosternal junction
C. floating ribs	F. body	I. suprasternal notch

1. _____ first seven pairs of ribs

2. _____ next five pairs of ribs

3. _____ last two pairs of false ribs

4. _____ lower tip of the sternum

5. _____ the ribs that are closest to the clavicle

6. _____ the depression on the superior border of the manubrium

7. _____ ribs that attach directly to the sternum by the costal cartilage

8. _____ the part of the sternum closest to the collarbone

9. _____ ribs that do not attach to the sternum

10. _____ ribs that attach indirectly to the sternum

11. _____ the largest part of the sternum; located between the manubrium and the xiphoid process

12. _____ the articulation between the manubrium and the body of the breastbone

13. _____ also called the *angle of Louis*

14. _____ rib #2 is located at this articulation

15. _____ should be less than 90 degrees

MATCHING

Bones Forming the Shoulder Girdle and Upper Extremities

Directions. Match the following terms to the most appropriate definition by writing the correct letter in the space provided. Some terms may be used more than once. See text pp. 121-122.

A. humerus
B. phalanges
C. glenoid cavity
D. scapula
E. ulna

F. pectoral girdle
G. carpals
H. pollux
I. acromion

J. metacarpals
K. olecranon process
L. radius
M. clavicle

1. _____ shoulder blade or wing bone

2. _____ depression where the head of the humerus articulates with the scapula

3. _____ long bone of the upper arm

4. _____ bony point of the ulna that forms the elbow

5. _____ collarbone

6. _____ bones that form the palm of the hand

7. _____ fourteen bones that form the fingers

8. _____ bone that contains the glenoid cavity

9. _____ the clavicle and scapula form this structure

10. _____ the scapula articulates with this bone to form a ball-and-socket joint at the shoulder

11. _____ the ulna and this bone articulate to form a hinge joint at the elbow

12. _____ bone that contains the olecranon fossa

13. _____ long bone in the lower arm that is located on the side of the little finger

14. _____ wrist bones

15. _____ bone in the lower arm that is on the thumb side

16. _____ pointy part of the shoulder

17. _____ also called the *shoulder girdle*

18. _____ the head of this bone articulates with the glenoid cavity

19. _____ contains the acromion and coracoid process

20. _____ bones that articulate with the proximal phalanges

21. _____ bone that contains the olecranon process

22. _____ the radius and this bone "cross" during supination

23. _____ long slender bone that articulates with both the sternum and the scapula

24. _____ the thumb

25. _____ the phalange that contains only two bones

Student Name _____

READ THE DIAGRAM

Shoulder and Upper Extremities

Directions. Refer to the diagram and write the numbers in the blanks. See text p. 123.

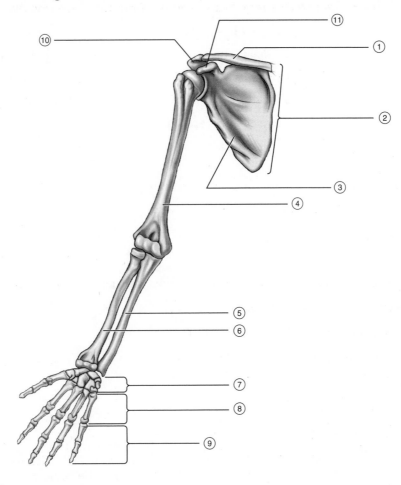

1. _____ scapula

2. _____ articulates with the ulna and scapula

3. _____ bone that contains the glenoid cavity

4. _____ the scapula articulates with this bone to form a ball-and-socket joint at the shoulder

5. _____ bone that contains the olecranon fossa

6. _____ ulna

7. _____ small bones that are distal to the radius and proximal to the metacarpals

8. _____ radius

9. _____ pectoral girdle

10. _____ the acromion

11. _____ coracoid process

12. _____ bone that contains the olecranon process

13. _____ the radius and this bone "cross" during supination

14. _____ long, slender bone that articulates with both the sternum and the scapula

MATCHING

Bones of the Pelvic Girdle and Lower Extremities

Directions. Match the following terms to the most appropriate definition by writing the correct letter in the space provided. Some terms may be used more than once. See text pp. 122-127.

A. coxal bone

B. symphysis pubis

C. trochanter

D. tibia

E. metatarsals

F. calcaneus

G. fibula

H. acetabulum

I. obturator

J. ilium

K. ischial tuberosity

L. patella

M. femur

N. pelvic girdle

O. phalanges

P. hallux

Q. talus

1. _____ the part of the coxal bone on which you sit

2. _____ bone that contains the obturator foramen

3. _____ kneecap

4. _____ shinbone

5. _____ cartilaginous disc between the two pubic bones; the disc expands during pregnancy

6. _____ the part of the hipbone that "flares"

7. _____ the instep of the foot is formed by these bones

8. _____ thin non–weight-bearing long bone of the leg

9. _____ heel bone

10. _____ bony process on the femur

11. _____ toes

12. _____ largest bone in the body; called the *thigh bone*

13. _____ the head of the femur articulates with this depression in the coxal bone

14. _____ the depression formed by the union of the ilium, ischium, and pubis

15. _____ formed by the two coxal bones

16. _____ the distal end of this bone is the lateral malleolus

17. _____ articulates with the coxal bone to form the hip and the tibia to form the knee

18. _____ the distal end of this bone is the medial malleolus

19. _____ composed of the pubis, ischium, and ilium

20. _____ the great toe

21. _____ this tarsal articulates with both the tibia and fibula

22. _____ the long weight-bearing bone in the leg

23. _____ forms the ball of the foot

24. _____ the two-bone phalange

Student Name _____

READ THE DIAGRAM

Hip and Lower Extremity

Directions. Refer to the diagram and then write the umbers in the blanks. See text pp. 125-126.

1. _____ patella

2. _____ shinbone

3. _____ the instep of the foot is formed by these bones

4. _____ thin nonweight-bearing long bone of the leg

5. _____ bony process on the femur

6. _____ phalanges

7. _____ largest bone in the body; called the *thigh bone*

8. _____ contains the ac-etabulum

9. _____ the distal end of this bone is the lateral malleolus

10. _____ articulates with the coxal bone to form the hip and the tibia to form the knee

11. _____ the distal end of this bone is the medial malleolus

12. _____ composed of the pubis, ischium, and ilium

13. _____ the long weight-bearing bone in the leg

MATCHING

Bone Markings

Directions. Indicate the bone on which each marking occurs. See text pp. 112-127.

A. femur

B. ulna

C. temporal

D. tibia

E. humerus

F. scapula

G. occipital

H. sternum

I. fibula

J. coxal

K. axis

L. sphenoid

1. _____ lateral malleolus

2. _____ foramen magnum

3. _____ zygomatic process

4. _____ medial malleolus

5. _____ greater sciatic notch

6. _____ obturator foramen

7. _____ olecranon process

8. _____ symphysis pubis

9. _____ greater trochanter

10. _____ acromion process

11. _____ external auditory meatus

12. _____ iliac crest

13. _____ olecranon fossa

14. _____ glenoid cavity

15. _____ acetabulum

16. _____ ischial tuberosity

17. _____ odentoid process ("dens")

18. _____ mastoid process

19. _____ sella turcica

20. _____ xiphoid process

21. _____ coracoid process

22. _____ lesser trochanter

23. _____ jugular notch

Student Name _____

MATCHING

Movement and Joints

Directions. Match the following terms to the most appropriate definition by writing the correct letter in the space provided. Some terms may be used more than once. See text pp. 127-133.

A. suture
B. ball-and-socket
C. flexion
D. hinge
E. pronation

F. supination
G. extension
H. slightly movable joints
I. dorsiflexion
J. adduction

K. circumduction
L. plantar flexion
M. abduction
N. bursae
O. ligament

1. _____ the type of freely movable joint at the elbow

2. _____ the type of joint formed by the acetabulum and the head of the femur

3. _____ the type of joint that connects the frontal and parietal bones

4. _____ small sacs of synovial fluid that ease movement at the joint

5. _____ the symphysis pubis and intervertebral discs, for example

6. _____ the type of joint formed by the head of the humerus and the glenoid cavity

7. _____ turning the forearm so that the palm is facing the sky

8. _____ describes the tiptoe position, relative to your foot

9. _____ describes bending the foot toward the shin

10. _____ the type of joint formed by the distal finger bones

11. _____ a circular type of movement made at a ball-and-socket joint such as the shoulder (as in pitching a softball)

12. _____ movement away from the midline of the body

13. _____ type of movement achieved as the lower arm bends toward the upper arm (decreasing the angle at the joint)

14. _____ tough strands of connective tissue that connect bone to bone

15. _____ straightening of a joint so that the angle between bones increases

16. _____ movement toward the midline of the body

17. _____ turning the forearm so that the hand is facing downward (toward the ground)

18. _____ example of an immovable joint

WRITE-IN

The Joints

Directions. Below is a list of joints. Draw a line to each joint on the skeleton and write the name of the joint on the line.

1. humeroulnar joint

2. tibiofibular joint (proximal)

3. manubriosternal (or sternomanubrial) joint

4. temporomandibular joint

5. sternoclavicular joint

6. acromioclavicular joint

7. humeroradial joint

8. metacarpophalangeal joint

9. tibiofemoral joint

10. symphysis pubis

11. glenohumeral joint

12. radiocarpal joint

13. tibiofibular joint (distal)

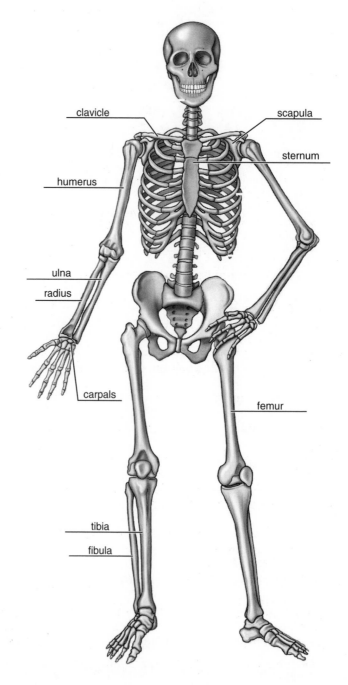

Student Name _____

READ THE DIAGRAM

The Skeleton

Directions. Referring to the illustration, fill in the blanks with the correct number.

1. _____ Bone that articulates with the radius and humerus.

2. _____ Bones that are distal to the radius and ulna and proximal to the metacarpals.

3. _____ Head of this large bone that articulates with the acetabulum of the coxal bone.

4. _____ Bone that is lateral to the tibia.

5. _____ Bones that are distal to the tibia and fibula and proximal to the metatarsals.

6. _____ Upper extremity phalanges.

7. _____ Bone that contains the "pointy" part of the elbow.

8. _____ Bone that is composed of the ilium, ischium, and pubis.

9. _____ The ulna and this bone supinate and pronate.

10. _____ Bone that is composed of the manubrium, body, and xiphoid process.

11. _____ Bone that contains the greater and lesser trochanter and articulates with the coxal bone.

12. _____ The scapula and this bone form the pectoral girdle.

13. _____ Bone that contains the glenoid cavity and allows ball-and-socket movement of the arm.

14. _____ Bone that is called the *wingbone*.

15. _____ Bone that contains the obturator foramen.

16. _____   Thigh bone; the largest bone in the body.

17. _____   The distal end of this bone is called the *lateral malleolus*.

18. _____   The distal end of this bone is called the *medial malleolus*.

19. _____   Bones that form the palms of the hands.

20. _____   The ulna and this bone form a hinge joint at the elbow.

21. _____   Long bone in the lower arm that is located on the "little finger" side of the arm.

22. _____   Talus.

READ THE DIAGRAM

The Skeleton

Directions. Referring the diagram (previous page) indicate the name of the bone and whether it is part of the appendicular or axial skeleton. Put the answers in the lines opposite the bone number (bone #12, the femur, appendicular skeleton, is done for you.)

Bone Number	Bone Name	Skeleton Part
#12	Femur	Appendicular
#15		
#6		
#16		
#13		
#24		
#21		
#19		
#3		
#7		
#14		
#25		
#4		
#20		

COLORING

The Skeleton

Directions. Refer to the illustration (p. 79 in the Study Guide). Color the bones according to the directions.

Red	phalanges
Yellow	metacarpals and metatarsals
Green	the bones that articulate with the femur
Blue	all bones that are distal to the glenoid cavity and proximal to the wrist
Black	sternum and true ribs
Orange	patella, calcaneus, mandible, and floating ribs

Student Name _____

READ THE DIAGRAM

Movements

Directions. Referring to the illustration, fill in the blanks with the words listed below.

A. flexion

B. extension

C. inversion

D. adduction

E. supination

F. eversion

G. circumduction

H. hyperextension

I. pronation

J. plantar flexion

K. dorsiflexion

L. abduction

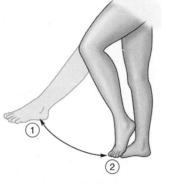
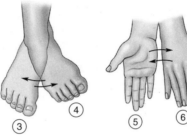
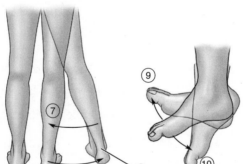
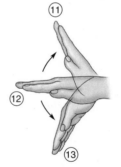
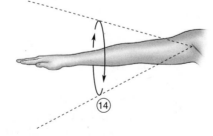

1. _____ movement from 1 → 2

2. _____ movement from 3 → 4

3. _____ movement from 5 → 6

4. _____ movement illustrated by #7

5. _____ movement from 9 → 10

6. _____ movement from 13 → 12

7. _____ movement from 12 → 11

8. _____ movement from 2 → 1

9. _____ movement from 4 → 3

10. _____ movement from 6 → 5

11. _____ movement illustrated by 8

12. _____ movement from 10 → 9

13. _____ movement from 11 → 13

14. _____ movement from 12 → 13

15. _____ movement illustrated by #14

READ THE DIAGRAM

Movements

*Directions. **Referring to the illustration on the previous page, fill in the number described below.***

1. _____ illustrates the pronated extremity

2. _____ illustrates the extremity in plantar flexion

3. _____ illustrates the everted extremity

4. _____ illustrates the movement of a ball-and-socket joint

5. _____ illustrates the effects of the crossing of the ulna and radius

6. _____ illustrates dorsiflexion of the extremity

7. _____ illustrates the movement of the lower extremity toward the midline on the body

8. _____ illustrates movement of the head of the humerus within the glenoid cavity

9. _____ illustrates movement of the head of the femur within the acetabulum; thigh abducts

PART II: PUTTING IT ALL TOGETHER

MULTIPLE CHOICE

*Directions. **Choose the correct answer.***

1. The purpose of the articular cartilage is to
    a. provide oxygenated blood to the osteon (haversian system).
    b. reduce friction within the joint.
    c. produce blood cells.
    d. act as a site of attachment for ligaments.

2. Injury to the epiphyseal disc is most likely to
    a. impair longitudinal bone growth.
    b. suppress blood cell formation causing anemia.
    c. cause bone softening and bowing of the legs.
    d. deprive the bone of oxygenated blood.

Student Name _____

3. Which of the following is true of the periosteum?

   a. lines the medullary cavities
   b. makes blood cells
   c. covers the outside of the diaphysis
   d. covers the distal end of long bones so as to minimize friction within the joints

4. Parathyroid hormone

   a. lowers blood levels of calcium.
   b. stimulates the bone marrow to make blood cells.
   c. stimulates bone formation.
   d. stimulates osteoclastic activity.

5. Which of the following is most likely to increase bone density?

   a. excess parathyroid hormone activity
   b. osteoblastic activity
   c. bone marrow depression
   d. prolonged bedrest

6. Which of the following is least true of the shoulder girdle?

   a. is also called the *pectoral girdle*
   b. includes the scapulae and clavicles
   c. supports the weight of the skull
   d. attaches the upper extremities to the axial skeleton

7. Which of the following is true of the femur?

   a. contains the olecranon process
   b. articulates with the coxal bone at the acetabulum
   c. articulates with both the coxal bone and the coccyx
   d. is also called the *shin bone*

8. The lateral malleolus and medial malleolus are located on the

   a. distal tibia.
   b. distal fibula.
   c. proximal and distal tibia.
   d. distal leg bones.

9. Which of the following is not characteristic of vertebrae?

   a. stacked in a column and separated by discs of cartilage
   b. include the atlas and axis
   c. include the sacrum and coccyx
   d. include the body, manubrium, and xiphoid process

10. Fontanels and unfused sutures in the infant skull

   a. are abnormal.
   b. allow for the expansion of the skull for brain growth.
   c. occur only in the presence of maternal deprivation of calcium.
   d. close and fuse within the first month.

11. The cranium

   a. contains all of the bones of the skull.
   b. includes the sphenoid, occipital bone, and the zygomatic bone.
   c. houses the brain.
   d. includes the occipital bone, the atlas, and the axis.

12. The occipital bone

   a. contains the obturator foramen.
   b. contains the foramen magnum.
   c. articulates with the cervical prominens.
   d. articulates with the parietal bones at the coronal suture.

13. The foramen magnum

   a. houses the pituitary gland.
   b. allows for the descent of the central nervous system as the spinal cord.
   c. is the site of attachment for the large thigh muscles.
   d. forms the eye sockets.

14. This patient has his mandible wired to his maxilla.

   a. an older adult patient who fell and broke his hip
   b. an infant with a developing hydrocephalus (expanding cranial circumference)
   c. an intoxicated young male with a fractured jaw
   d. a middle-aged male with an abscessed tooth

15. The temporal bone

   a. is a facial bone.
   b. contains the mastoid, styloid, and zygomatic processes.
   c. articulates with the maxilla at the TMJ.
   d. contains the foramen magnum.

16. The ulna

    a. articulates with the scapula at the glenoid cavity.
    b. forms a ball-and-socket joint with the radius.
    c. forms a hinge joint with the humerus.
    d. articulates with the tarsals to form the wrist.

17. Which of the following supinate and pronate?

    a. scapula and clavicle
    b. manubrium and xiphoid process
    c. femur and tibia
    d. ulna and radius

18. Which of the following are aligned parallel to each other?

    a. femur and tibia
    b. tibia and calcaneus
    c. fibula and patella
    d. tibia and fibula

19. The acetabulum

    a. is located on the femur.
    b. is formed by the ilium, ischium, and pubis.
    c. is part of the axial skeleton.
    d. forms the knee.

20. Which of the following is not part of the knee?

    a. distal femur
    b. patella
    c. proximal tibia
    d. acetabulum

21. This guy is a heel!

    a. Phil Anges
    b. Cal C. Aneus
    c. Max Illa
    d. Hugh Merus

22. Mr. Phil Anges was named after

    a. his fingers and toes.
    b. a mountain in South America.
    c. a Gucci glove.
    d. his thermal socks.

CASE STUDY

T.B., a 65-year-old woman, fell as she was leaving her home. She was unable to move her left leg and appeared to be in extreme pain when the paramedics transported her to a litter. She was later diagnosed with a fractured hip and sent to surgery where a pin was inserted into the fractured bone. A bone scan indicated a decrease in bone density.

1. Which anatomical structure was fractured?

    a. iliac crest of the coxal bone
    b. ischial tuberosity of the hip bone
    c. greater trochanter of the femur
    d. neck of the femur

2. Where was the trochanter roll placed after surgery?

    a. over the abdomen of the patient to provide privacy
    b. partially under and alongside the affected thigh to prevent an outward rotation of the hip
    c. at the sole of the foot to prevent plantar flexion
    d. under the coccyx to align the hip with the lower back

3. Given her age and medical history, what does the decrease in her bone density suggest?

    a. cancer of the bone
    b. osteoporosis
    c. congenital defect of the bone
    d. infection of the bone

Student Name _____

PART III: CHALLENGE YOURSELF!

GROUPS AND PUZZLE

1. Which group is incorrect?

    a. bones of the lower extremities: femur, tibia, sternum
    b. types of freely movable joints: hinge, ball-and-socket
    c. bones of the axial skeleton: sternum, vertebrae, ribs
    d. types of movement: flexion, pronation, abduction

2. Which group is incorrect?

    a. spinal curvatures: cervical, thoracic, lumbar, sacral
    b. abnormal curvatures of the spine: scoliosis, kyphosis, lordosis
    c. types of ribs: true, false, floating
    d. bones of the upper extremities: humerus, radius, sternum

3. Which group is incorrect?

    a. types of bones: long, short, flat, irregular
    b. long bones: humerus, femur, tibia
    c. bones of the skull: frontal, parietal, temporal, atlas
    d. sinuses: frontal, maxillary, sphenoidal, ethmoidal

PUZZLE

Hint: Personal Brain Bucket

Directions. Perform the following functions on the Sequence of Words below. When all functions have been performed, you are left with a word(s) related to the hint.

Functions: remove the following:

1. all vertebral bones (3)

2. bones that form the acetabulum (3)

3. bones that form the pectoral girdle (2)

4. bones of the lower extremity (7)

5. facial bones (4)

6. bones in the arm, wrist, and palm of the hand (5)

Sequence of Words

ILIUMHUMERUSETHMOIDFIBULAMANDIBLECARPALSATLASMAXILLAISCHIUMCLAVI
CLEMETACARPALSSACRUMULNAZYGOMATICMETATARSALSPUBISTIBIASCAPULAPHA
LANGESFEMURRADIUSTARSALSAXISPATELLACRANIUM

Answer: _____

BODY TOONS

Hint: an Indonesian volcano

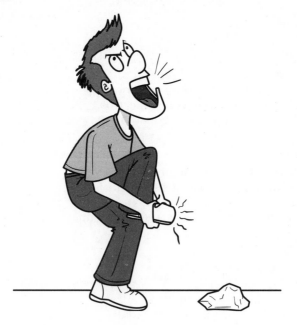

Hint: Name this bone in the appendicular zone.

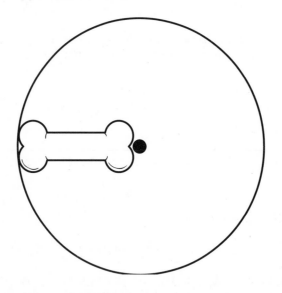

9

Muscular System

Answer Key: Textbook page references are provided as a guide for answering these questions. A complete answer key was provided for your instructor.

Objectives

1. Identify three types of muscle tissue.

2. Describe the sliding filament hypothesis of muscle contraction.

3. Describe the events that occur at the neuromuscular junction.

4. Explain the role of calcium and adenosine triphosphate in muscle contraction.

5. Identify the sources of energy for muscle contraction.

6. Trace the sequence of events from nerve stimulation to muscle contraction.

7. Define twitch, tetanus, and recruitment.

8. State the basis for naming muscles.

9. List the actions of the major muscles.

PART I: MASTERING THE BASICS

MATCHING

Types of Muscle

Directions. Match the following terms to the most appropriate definition by writing the correct letter in the space provided. Some terms may be used more than once. See text pp. 138-139.

A. skeletal muscle

B. smooth muscle

C. cardiac muscle

1. _____ striated and voluntary

2. _____ found in the walls of organs or viscera

3. _____ found in the walls of blood vessels

4. _____ striated and involuntary

5. _____ found in the heart

6. _____ nonstriated and involuntary

7. _____ found attached to bones

8. _____ the only type of muscle that is nonstriated

9. _____ the only type of muscle that is voluntary

10. _____ must be supplied by a motor nerve

MATCHING

Parts of a Whole Muscle

Directions. Match the following terms to the most appropriate definition by writing the correct letter in the space provided. Some terms may be used more than once. See text p. 139.

A. fascicles

B. perimysium

C. endomysium

D. aponeurosis

E. tendon

F. epimysium

1. _____ cordlike structure that attaches muscle to bone

2. _____ small bundles of muscle fibers

3. _____ connective tissue that surrounds individual muscle fibers

4. _____ flat, sheetlike fascia that attaches muscle to muscle or muscle to bone

5. _____ connective tissue that surrounds the fascicles or bundles

6. _____ connective tissue that surrounds a whole skeletal muscle

Student Name _____

MATCHING

Structure of a Muscle Fiber

Directions. Match the following terms to the most appropriate definition by writing the correct letter in the space provided. See text pp. 139-141.

A. T tubule

C. actin

E. myosin

B. sarcoplasmic reticulum (SR)

D. sarcomere

F. cross-bridge

1. _____   series of contractile units that make up each myofibril; extends from Z line to Z line

2. _____   thin protein filaments that extend toward the center of the sarcomere from the Z lines

3. _____   thick protein filaments whose "heads" form cross-bridges when they interact with the thin filaments

4. _____   calcium is stored within this structure in the relaxed muscle

5. _____   an extension of the sarcolemma or cell membrane that penetrates into the interior of the muscle; the electrical signal runs along this membrane toward the sarcoplasmic reticulum

6. _____   the temporary connection formed when the myosin heads interact with the actin, causing muscle contraction

ORDERING

Muscle Stimulation, Contraction, and Relaxation

Directions. Using numbers 1 to 8, place the following events in the correct order. The first and fourth events are labeled for you. See text pp. 140-144.

_____   The electrical signal (nerve impulse) causes the vesicles within the nerve terminal to fuse with the membrane and release the neurotransmitter acetylcholine (ACh).

_____   Muscle relaxation occurs when calcium is pumped back into the sarcoplasmic reticulum.

_____   The electrical signal in the muscle membrane travels along the sarcolemma (muscle membrane) and penetrates deep into the muscle by the T tubular system.

____4____   ACh stimulates the receptors and causes an electrical signal to develop along the muscle membrane.

____1____   Stimulation of the motor nerve causes an electrical signal to move along the somatic nerve toward the nerve ending.

_____   The calcium allows the actin, myosin, and ATP to form cross-bridges, thereby causing muscle contraction.

_____   ACh diffuses across the junction and binds to the receptor sites on the muscle membrane.

_____   The electrical signal stimulates the sarcoplasmic reticulum to release calcium into the sarcomere area.

MATCHING

Muscle Terms

Directions. Match the following terms to the most appropriate definition by writing the correct letter in the space provided. Some terms may be used more than once. See text p. 146.

A. origin

B. insertion

C. antagonist

D. hypertrophy

E. synergist

F. prime mover

G. atrophy

H. contracture

1. _____ the muscle responsible for most of the movement in a group of muscles; called the *chief muscle*

2. _____ muscle attachment to the movable bone

3. _____ an increase in the size of a muscle due to overuse

4. _____ muscle attachment to the stationary bone

5. _____ helper muscle; it works with other muscles to produce the same movement

6. _____ abnormal formation of fibrous tissue in muscles, preventing normal mobility

7. _____ muscle that opposes the action of another muscle

8. _____ wasting away or decrease in the size of the muscles

MATCHING

Naming Skeletal Muscles

Directions. Match the following terms to the most appropriate definition by writing the correct letter in the space provided. Some terms may be used more than once. See text pp. 146-147.

A. vastus

B. deltoid

C. brevis

D. rectus

E. pectoralis

F. brachii

G. gluteus

H. maximus

I. teres

J. latissimus

K. oblique

1. _____ short

2. _____ diagonal

3. _____ triangular

4. _____ round

5. _____ buttock

6. _____ large

7. _____ huge

8. _____ arm

9. _____ wide

10. _____ straight

11. _____ chest

Student Name _____

MATCHING

Muscles of the Head and Neck

Directions. Match the following terms to the most appropriate definition by writing the correct letter in the space provided. Some terms may be used more than once. See text pp. 147-153.

A. frontalis   D. buccinator   G. sternocleidomastoid

B. orbicularis oculi   E. masseter   H. zygomaticus

C. orbicularis oris   F. temporalis   I. trapezius

1. _____ muscle that flattens the cheek when contracted; it positions food for chewing

2. _____ flat muscle that raises the eyebrows and wrinkles the forehead; creates a surprised look

3. _____ fan-shaped muscle that extends from the temporal bone to the mandible; it works synergistically with other chewing muscles

4. _____ extends from the corners of the mouth to the cheekbone; called the *smiling muscle*

5. _____ muscle of the upper back and neck. Contraction of this muscle tilts the head so that the face looks up at the sky; also moves the shoulder

6. _____ sphincter muscle encircling the mouth; called the *kissing muscle*

7. _____ muscles on either side of the neck that cause flexion of the head as in praying; contraction of only one of these muscles rotates the head

8. _____ a chewing muscle that works synergistically with the temporalis muscle to close the jaw

9. _____ sphincter muscle encircling the eyes; assists in winking, blinking, and squinting

10. _____ works antagonistically to the sternocleidomastoid

11. _____ a spasm of this muscle causes torticollis, or wryneck

12. _____ attaches to the collar bone, breast bone, and temporal bone

MATCHING

Muscles of the Trunk and Extremities

Directions. Match the following terms to the most appropriate definition by writing the correct letter in the space provided. Some terms may be used more than once. See text pp. 148-157.

A. intercostals

B. abdominal muscles

C. linea alba

D. adductors

E. triceps brachii

F. sartorius

G. trapezius

H. serratus anterior

I. hamstrings

J. pectoralis major

K. biceps brachii

L. quadriceps femoris

M. latissimus dorsi

N. gastrocnemius

O. gluteus maximus

P. deltoid

Q. diaphragm

R. tibialis anterior

S. soleus

1. _____ dome-shaped muscle that separates the thoracic cavity from the abdominal cavity

2. _____ the chief muscle of inhalation (breathing in)

3. _____ longest muscle in the body that is used to sit crossed-legged (lotus position)

4. _____ muscle that shrugs the shoulders and moves the head

5. _____ barbecued ribs

6. _____ jagged muscle that resembles the teeth of a saw; it lowers the shoulder and moves the arm, as in pushing a cart

7. _____ includes the internal oblique, external oblique, transversus, and rectus

8. _____ muscles located on the medial (inner) surface of the thigh; horseback riders use these muscles to grip the horse with their thighs

9. _____ group of muscles that extend or straighten the leg at the knee, as in kicking a football

10. _____ large, broad muscle located over the middle and lower back; it lowers the shoulders and brings the arms back, as in swimming and rowing

11. _____ the Achilles tendon attaches the soleus and this muscle to the heel bone

12. _____ large, broad muscle that forms the anterior chest wall; it connects the humerus with the clavicle and structures of the chest

13. _____ muscle that forms the shoulder pads; positions the arms in a "scarecrow" position

14. _____ muscles responsible for raising and lowering the rib cage during breathing

15. _____ a white line that extends from the sternum to the pubic bone; it is formed by the aponeurosis of the abdominal muscles on opposite sides of the abdomen

16. _____ muscle that flexes the forearm; when you ask a child to "make a muscle," this is the one that pops up

17. _____ muscle that lies along the posterior surface of the humerus; it extends the forearm and is used to bear weight in crutch-walking

18. _____ largest muscle in the body that forms part of the buttocks; you sit on this muscle

19. _____ the calf muscle that is used in plantar flexion; also called the *toe-dancer's muscle*

20. _____ muscle group on the posterior surface of the thigh that flexes the leg at the knee; antagonist to the quadriceps femoris

21. _____ works synergistically with the gastrocnemius

Student Name _____

22. _____ includes the rectus femoris and vastus lateralis

23. _____ located over the shin bone; causes dorsiflexion

24. _____ includes the biceps femoris

25. _____ the brachialis and the brachioradialis work synergistically with this muscle to flex the arm at the elbow

READ THE DIAGRAM

Muscles: Anterior View

Directions. Referring to the diagram (see text Figure 9-7, A, p. 148), fill in the spaces with the names of the muscles. Some muscles may be used more than once. See text pp. 148-151.

1. _____ the smiling muscle; extends from the corners of the mouth to the cheek-bone

2. _____ long muscle that lies obliquely over the anterior thigh; tailor's muscle; sitting cross-legged

3. _____ wrinkles forehead, raises eyebrows, gives a "surprised" look

4. _____ flexes and rotates the head; the "praying muscle"

5. _____ the major anterior chest muscle; adducts and flexes the upper arm across the chest

6. _____ the white line of the abdomen; extends from the sternum to the pubic bone

7. _____ an abdominal muscle; fibers runs vertically from the sternum to the pubic bone

8. _____ an abdominal muscle; fibers run horizontally

9. _____ shoulder pad; "scarecrow" position of the arms

10. _____ works synergistically with the brachialis and brachioradialis to flex and supinate the forearm

11. _____ includes the rectus femoris, vastus lateralis, and vastus medialis

12. _____ a muscle group that "kicks" a football; it extends the leg

13. _____ causes dorsiflexion of the foot

14. _____ the temporalis and this muscle are the chewing muscles

15. _____ the adductor magnus and this muscle move the thigh towards the mid-line of the body

16. _____ a circular muscle that causes winking, blinking, and squinting

17. _____ sites of attachment: clavicle, temporal bone, and breastbone

18. _____ spasm of this muscle causes torticollis

19. _____ a jagged muscle that lies along the lateral chest wall

READ THE DIAGRAM

Muscles: Posterior View

Directions. Referring to the diagram (see text Figure 9-7, B), fill in the spaces with the names of the muscles. Some muscles may be used more than once. See text pp. 149-151.

1. _____ extends the head (allows the face to look at the sky); attached to the base of the occipital bone and the spines of the upper vertebral column

2. _____ lies along the posterior humerus; extends the forearm; the "boxer's muscle"

3. _____ your big "sitting muscle;" largest muscle in the body

4. _____ this group includes the biceps femoris, semitendinosus, semimembranosus

5. _____ the soleus and this muscle cause plantar flexion

6. _____ a large, broad muscle located across the middle and lower back; called the *swimmer's muscle*

7. _____ lies along the posterior humerus; bears most of the body weight during crutch-walking

8. _____ this muscle group is antagonistic to the quadriceps femoris group

9. _____ the strong tendons of this muscle group can be felt behind the knee (gives rise to the name of this group)

10. _____ the gastrocnemius and this muscle are called the *toe-dancer's muscle*

11. _____ the calf muscles attach to this tendon; the tendon attaches to the heel bone

PART II: PUTTING IT ALL TOGETHER

MULTIPLE CHOICE

Directions. Choose the correct answer.

1. Which muscles produce movement of the extremities, maintain body posture, and stabilize joints?

   a. smooth muscle
   b. muscles that are nonstriated and involuntary
   c. skeletal muscles
   d. striated muscles that are involuntary

2. Which muscles are found in the bronchioles (breathing passages) and the blood vessels?

   a. skeletal muscle
   b. muscle that is striated and voluntary
   c. smooth muscle
   d. muscle that is striated and involuntary

Student Name _____

3. Which structures slide in the sliding filament hypothesis of muscle contraction?

   a. T tubules and the sarcoplasmic reticulum
   b. actin and myosin
   c. calcium and ATP
   d. epimysium and the perimysium

4. What is the consequence of recruitment?

   a. paralysis
   b. increased force of muscle contraction
   c. depletion of acetylcholine in the neuro-muscular junction
   d. inability of the muscle to contract

5. What is the role of the sarcoplasmic reticulum (SR) is muscle contraction?

   a. synthesizes actin
   b. synthesizes myosin
   c. releases calcium into the sarcomere
   d. releases acetylcholine (ACh) into the neuromuscular junction

6. What is the consequence of tetanus?

   a. muscles twitching
   b. flaccid paralysis
   c. sustained muscle contraction
   d. atrophy

7. What happens when receptor sites on the muscle membrane are damaged so that the transmitter ACh cannot bind properly?

   a. The muscle hypertrophies.
   b. Muscle contraction is impaired and the patient experiences muscle weakness.
   c. The muscle tetanizes.
   d. The skeletal muscle loses its striations and becomes a smooth muscle.

8. What event causes the muscle to relax?

   a. Calcium is pumped back into the sarco-plasmic reticulum.
   b. ATP is pumped into the sarcoplasmic reticulum.
   c. The muscle becomes depleted of actin.
   d. The muscle becomes depleted of myosin.

9. What happens when you repetitively and rapidly stimulate a skeletal muscle?

   a. the muscle delivers a single twitch
   b. a flaccid paralysis develops
   c. the muscle tetanizes
   d. the muscle "freezes" and develops a contracture

10. Which of the following terminates events in the neuromuscular junction?

    a. Calcium is pumped back into the nerve terminal.
    b. The receptors are blocked with actin.
    c. The receptors are blocked with myosin cross-bridges.
    d. Acetylcholine is inactivated.

11. What action is antagonistic to the biceps brachii muscle?

    a. The brachialis contracts.
    b. The deltoid contracts.
    c. The triceps brachii contracts.
    d. The brachioradialis contracts.

12. Which condition is most likely to develop in a person whose leg is in a nonweight-bearing cast for several months?

    a. disuse muscle atrophy of the affected leg
    b. hypertrophy of the affected leg
    c. compression of the growth plate causing the affected leg to be shorter than normal
    d. osteoporosis and pathologic fractures

13. Which of the following is indicated by the terms *pectoralis, gluteus, brachii,* and *lateralis?*

    a. location of a muscle
    b. shape of a muscle
    c. size of a muscle
    d. muscle action

14. Which of the following is indicated by the terms *biceps, triceps,* and *quadriceps?*

    a. numbers of origins of the muscle
    b. direction of fibers of the muscle
    c. shape of the muscle
    d. muscle action

15. What is the basis for naming the sternocleido-mastoid muscle?

    a. sites of attachment of the muscle
    b. shape of the muscle
    c. size of the muscle
    d. muscle action

16. The hamstrings

    a. extend the leg at the knee (as in kicking a football).
    b. are located on the posterior thigh.
    c. work synergistically with the quadriceps group to adduction the leg.
    d. flex the thigh at the hip.

17. Rigor mortis develops
    a. only in smooth muscle.
    b. in response to a depletion of calcium in the sarcomere.
    c. in response to a buildup of lactic acid and creatine phosphate.
    d. in response to a deficiency of ATP.

18. Creatine phosphate
    a. is an energy source for muscle contraction.
    b. is a contractile protein.
    c. forms the cross-bridges between actin and myosin.
    d. inactivates acetylcholine within the neuromuscular junction.

19. Which of the following is least descriptive of the deltoid muscle?
    a. forms shoulder pads
    b. is a common site of injection of drugs
    c. elevates the arm to a scarecrow position
    d. has its origin on the humerus

20. Why may the weight of bed linen on a bedridden patient cause a disabling contracture?
    a. The linen causes a prolonged dorsiflexion.
    b. The linen adducts the leg.
    c. The linen forces the foot into a position of plantar flexion.
    d. The linen compresses the nerve that supplies the muscles of the feet

21. Which condition is most associated with aging?
    a. conversion of skeletal muscle to smooth muscle
    b. gradual loss of muscle strength
    c. an overproduction of myoglobin
    d. conversion of smooth muscle to aponeurosis

22. Which of the following is most related to the role of myoglobin?
    a. muscle contraction
    b. synthesis of actin and myosin
    c. storage of calcium
    d. carrier of oxygen

23. Supinators and pronators
    a. are types of smooth muscle.
    b. have their origin on the scapula.
    c. twist the lower arm.
    d. flex the fingers.

CASE STUDY

B.J. was scheduled for abdominal surgery. In addition to the general anesthetics, B.J. was also given a curare-like drug during surgery.

1. What was the purpose of the curare-like drug?
    a. cause sedation
    b. deaden or numb the entire abdomen
    c. cause muscle relaxation
    d. cause unconsciousness

2. Why may the curare-like drug affect respirations? It
    a. depresses the respiratory center in the brain.
    b. binds or inactivates oxygen.
    c. interferes with activity in the neuromuscular junction, thereby impairing contraction of the respiratory muscles.
    d. causes swelling of the tongue and cuts off the flow of air into the lungs.

Student Name _____

PART III: CHALLENGE YOURSELF!

GROUPS AND PUZZLE

1. Which group is incorrect?

   a. types of muscles: skeletal, smooth, cardiac
   b. types of striated muscle: skeletal, smooth, cardiac
   c. muscles involved in breathing: diaphragm, intercostals
   d. muscles in the upper extremities: biceps brachii, triceps brachii, supinators

2. Which group is incorrect?

   a. contractile proteins: actin, myosin
   b. types of connective tissue: tendons, perimysium, aponeurosis
   c. movements: flexion, supination, abduction
   d. types of involuntary muscles: skeletal, smooth, cardiac

3. Which group is incorrect?

   a. muscles in the upper part of the body: deltoid, biceps brachii, hamstrings
   b. movements: flexion, supination, abduction
   c. muscles in lower extremities: hamstrings, quadriceps femoris, gastrocnemius
   d. contractile proteins: actin, myosin

PUZZLE

Hint $\dfrac{\textbf{Muscle}}{\text{Use}}$, $\dfrac{\textbf{Use}}{\text{Muscle}}$

Directions. Perform the following functions on the Sequence of Words below. When all the functions have been performed, you are left with word(s) that are related to the hint. Record your answer below.

Functions: remove the following

1. muscle group on the anterior thigh; muscle group on the posterior thigh
2. tendon that attaches the gastrocnemius to the calcaneus
3. muscle that causes plantar flexion
4. transmitter within the neuromuscular junction
5. muscles (2) of mastication
6. muscle terms that mean *round, triangular, short,* and *diagonal*
7. muscle that attaches to the temporal bone, sternum, and clavicle
8. muscles that lie along the anterior upper arm and posterior upper arm
9. from Z line to Z line
10. muscle response to death

Sequence of Words

DELTOIDMASSETERSTERNOCLEIDOMASTOIDSARCOMEREGASTROCNEMIUSOBLIQU
EQUADRICEPSFEMORISACETYLCHOLINERIGORMORTISACHILLESTENDONATROPHYTRI
CEPSBRACHIIBICEPSBRACHIIHAMSTRINGSBREVISHYPERTROPHYTEMPORALISTERES

Answer _____, _____

Nervous System: Nervous Tissue and Brain

Answer Key: Textbook page references are provided as a guide for answering these questions. A complete answer key was provided for your instructor.

Objectives

1. Define the two divisions of the nervous system.

2. List three general functions of the nervous system.

3. Compare the structure and functions of the neuroglia and neuron.

4. Explain the function of the myelin sheath.

5. Explain how a neuron transmits information.

6. Describe the structure and function of a synapse

7. Describe the functions of the four major areas of the brain.

8. Describe the functions of the four lobes of the cerebrum.

9. Describe how the skull, meninges, cerebrospinal fluid, and blood-brain barrier protect the central nervous system.

PART I: MASTERING THE BASICS

✳ MATCHING

Organization of the Nervous System

Directions. Match the following terms to the most appropriate definition by writing the correct letter in the space provided. Some terms may be used more than once. See text p. 162.

A. central nervous system (CNS)

B. peripheral nervous system

C. motor nerves

D. sensory nerves

E. integrative function

1. __C__   nerves that carry out the plans made by the CNS

2. __A__   part of the nervous system that contains the brain and the spinal cord

3. __D__   also described as *afferent nerves*

4. __D__   nerves that gather information from the environment and carry it to the CNS

5. __B__   part of the nervous system consisting of nerves that connect the brain and the spinal cord with the rest of the body

6. __C__   also described as *efferent nerves*

7. __E__   the processing and interpretation of information by the cells of the CNS; the decision-making capability

MATCHING

Nerve Cells

Directions. Match the following terms to the most appropriate definition by writing the correct letter in the space provided. See text pp. 162-165.

A. neurons

B. astrocyte

C. ependymal cell

D. Schwann cells

E. ganglia

F. nuclei

G. microglia

H. neuroglia (glia)

1. __B__   common type of glial cell that supports and protects the neurons; the cell helps form the blood-brain barrier

2. __H__   nerve tissue that is called *nerve glue;* composed of astrocytes, microglia, oligodendrocytes, and ependymal cells

3. __A__   nerve cells that transmit information as electrical signals

4. __C__   type of glial cell that lines the inside cavities of the brain and helps form the cerebrospinal fluid

5. __G__   glial cells that engage in phagocytosis of pathogens and damaged tissue

6. __D__   glial cells that form the myelin sheath in the peripheral nervous system

7. __F__   clusters of cell bodies located within the CNS

8. __E__   clusters of cell bodies located in the peripheral nervous system

Student Name _____

MATCHING

Parts of a Neuron

Directions. Match the following terms to the most appropriate definition by writing the correct letter in the space provided. Some terms may be used more than once. See text pp. 164-165.

A. cell body

B. axon

C. axon terminal

D. nodes of Ranvier

E. neurilemma

F. myelin sheath

G. dendrites

H. acetylcholine

1. __B__ part of the neuron that transmits information away from the cell body

2. __A__ part of the neuron that contains the nucleus; dendrites bring information to this structure, and the axon carries information away from this structure

3. __F__ white, fatty material that surrounds the axon; it increases the rate at which the electrical signal travels along the axon

4. __D__ short segments of the axonal membrane that are not covered by myelin sheath

5. __C__ part of the axon where the neurotransmitters are stored

6. __G__ treelike part of the neuron that receives information from another neuron and transmits that information toward the cell body

7. __E__ a layer of cells that covers the axons of peripheral neurons; concerned with nerve regeneration

8. __F__ makes white matter white

9. __D__ allows for saltatory conduction of the nerve impulse

10. __H__ a common neurotransmitter

READE THE DIAGRAM

✳ Two Neurons and a Synapse

Directions. Referring to the illustration, write the numbers in the blanks. See text p. 170.

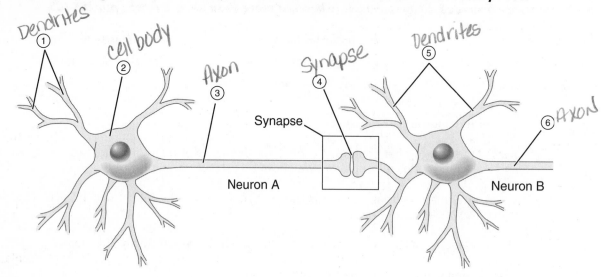

1. __2__ the cell body of neuron A
2. __6__ the axon of neuron B
3. __4__ the synapse
4. __5__ the dendrites of neuron B
5. __3__ the axon of neuron A
6. __1__ the dendrites of neuron A

COLORING AND DRAWING

Directions. For the figure above, color the appropriate areas as indicated below.

1. Color the dendrites of neuron A *red.*
2. Color the axon of neuron B *yellow.*
3. Color the presynaptic membrane *blue.*
4. Color the postsynaptic membrane *green.*

DRAW IN

Directions. For the figure above, draw in the structures indicated below.

1. the storage of the neurotransmitter within the vesicles of the axon terminal
2. the myelin sheath and nodes of Ranvier on the axon of neuron A
3. an arrow that indicates the direction of movement of the nerve impulse (action potential)

Student Name _____

MATCHING

Nerve Impulse

Directions. Match the following terms to the most appropriate definition by writing the correct letter in the space provided. Some terms may be used more than once. See text pp. 166-170.

A. depolarization
B. resting membrane potential (RMP)
C. refractory period
D. repolarization
E. action potential

1. __A__ the inside of the neuron becomes positively charged
2. __B__ the inside of the unstimulated neuron is negative; this electrical charge is caused by the outward leak of potassium (K⁺)
3. __D__ the depolarized neuron returns to the resting state
4. __A__ the first phase of the action potential caused by an inward movement of sodium (Na⁺)
5. __C__ the inability of a depolarized neuron to accept a stimulus until it has repolarized
6. __E__ the changes in electrical charge across the membrane during depolarization and repolarization; also called the *nerve impulse*
7. __D__ the second phase of the action potential that is caused by the outward movement of potassium (K⁺)

MATCHING

Bumps and Grooves

Directions. Match the following terms to the most appropriate definition by writing the correct letter in the space provided. Some terms may be used more than once. See text pp. 171-173.

A. central sulcus
B. sulcus
C. fissure
D. lateral sulcus
E. gyrus
F. precentral gyrus
G. postcentral gyrus
H. longitudinal fissure

1. __F__ convolution located on the frontal lobe immediately anterior to the central sulcus
2. __E__ a bump or elevation on the surface of the cerebrum
3. __B__ a shallow groove found on the surface of the brain
4. __C__ a deep groove found on the surface of the brain
5. __E__ also called a *convolution*
6. __G__ convolution that is located on the parietal lobe immediately posterior to the central sulcus
7. __A__ sulcus that separates the frontal lobe from the parietal lobes
8. __D__ groove that separates the temporal lobe from the frontal and parietal lobes
9. __H__ deep groove that separates the left and right hemispheres
10. __A__ sulcus that separates the primary motor cortex from the primary somatosensory cortex

MATCHING

✳ ## Parts of the Brain

Directions. Match the following terms to the most appropriate definition by writing the correct letter in the space provided. Some terms may be used more than once. See text pp. 172-178.

A. cerebrum	F. frontal lobe	K. occipital lobe
B. brain stem	G. parietal lobe	L. hypothalamus
C. diencephalon	H. temporal lobe	M. thalamus
D. pons	I. limbic system	N. medulla oblongata
E. cerebellum	J. reticular formation	O. corpus callosum

1. __A__ largest part of the brain

2. __I__ called the *emotional brain*

3. __M__ we first become aware of pain at this level of the diencephalon; however, this structure does not allow us to determine the kind of pain or to locate the source of the pain

4. __N__ part of the brain stem that connects the brain to the spinal cord

5. __G__ the central sulcus separates the frontal lobe from this lobe

6. __B__ composed of the midbrain, pons, and medulla oblongata

7. __L__ part of the diencephalon that controls the pituitary gland; it also helps control the autonomic nervous system, water balance, and body temperature

8. __A__ part of the brain that is divided into the right and left hemispheres

9. __C__ composed of the thalamus and the hypothalamus

10. __D__ this structure means *bridge;* it helps regulate breathing rate and rhythm

11. __O__ bands of white matter that join the right and left cerebral hemispheres

12. __F__ the precentral gyrus of this cerebral lobe is the major motor cortex; nerve impulses that originate in the motor area control voluntary muscle activity

13. __G__ the postcentral gyrus of this cerebral lobe is the primary somatosensory area

14. __F__ plays a key role in personality development, emotional and behavioral expression, and the performance of high-level thinking and learning tasks

15. __H__ cerebral lobe that contains the auditory cortex (hearing) and the olfactory area (smell)

16. __N__ part of the brain stem called the *vital center* because it regulates vital processes such as blood pressure, heart rate, and respirations

17. __N__ part of the brain stem that contains the vomiting center

18. __F__ cerebral lobe that contains the frontal eye fields

Student Name _____

19. __F__   cerebral lobe that controls motor speech

20. __N__   decussation of most motor fibers occurs here

21. __F__   a motor homunculus lives here

22. __G__   a sensory homunculus lives here

23. __K__   cerebral lobe that is primarily concerned with vision

24. __M__   part of the diencephalon that acts as a relay and sorting station for most sensory fibers

25. __J__   this widespread group of cells is concerned with the sleep/wake cycle and consciousness; signals passing from this structure to the cerebral cortex keep us awake

26. __F__   cerebral lobe that contains Broca's area

27. __K__   damage to this cerebral lobe causes cortical blindness

28. __N__   part of the brain stem that contains the emetic center

29. __E__   brain structure that protrudes from under the occipital lobe and is concerned primarily with the coordination of skeletal muscle activity

30. __H__   damage to this cerebral lobe causes cortical deafness

31. __N__   part of the brain stem that receives information from the chemoreceptor trigger zone (CTZ)

READ THE DIAGRAM

✴ Brain

Directions. Referring to the diagram, fill in the space with the correct numbers. See text pp. 172-178.

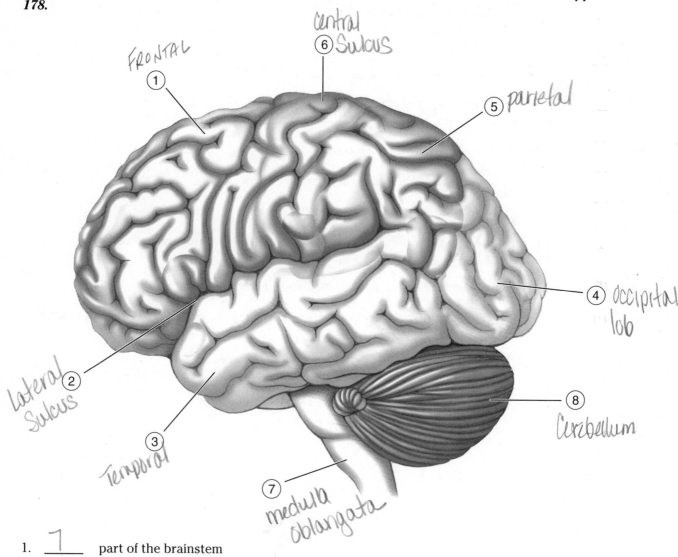

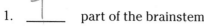

1. __7__   part of the brainstem

2. __7__   called the *vital center* because it regulates respirations, blood pressure, and heart rate

3. __5__   central sulcus that separates the frontal lobe from this lobe

4. __1__   the precentral gyrus of this cerebral lobe is the major motor cortex

5. __5__   the postcentral gyrus of this cerebral lobe is the primary somatosensory area

6. __6__   fissure or groove that separates the primary motor cortex from the primary somatosensory area

7. __4__   cerebral lobe that is concerned primarily with vision

Student Name _____

8. __3__ cerebral lobe that is concerned primarily with hearing

9. __1__ the lateral sulcus separates the temporal lobe from this anterior cerebral lobe

10. __1__ this cerebral lobe contains Broca's area

11. __8__ this "little brain" protrudes from under the occipital lobe and is concerned with skeletal muscle coordination

12. __1__ the pyramidal tract arises from this cerebral lobe; the tract carries electrical signals to skeletal muscles causing voluntary muscle contraction

13. __4__ destruction of this cerebral lobe causes cortical blindness

14. __3__ destruction of this cerebral lobe causes cortical deafness

15. __2__ this sulcus separates the frontal and parietal lobes from the temporal lobe

16. __7__ contains the emetic center

COLORING

Xs and Os...Yap Yap Yap

Directions. Color or mark the appropriate areas on the illustration on the previous page as indicated below.

1. Color the frontal lobe ***red.***
2. Color the occipital lobe ***yellow.***
3. Color the parietal lobe ***green.***
4. Color the temporal lobe ***blue.***
5. Put ***Xs*** in the precentral gyrus.
6. Put ***Os*** in the postcentral gyrus.
7. Label Broca's area as ***Yap Yap Yap.***
8. Put an ***E*** on the frontal eye fields.

MATCHING

Protection of the Brain and Spinal Cord

Directions. Match the following terms to the most appropriate definition by writing the correct letter in the space provided. See text pp. 178-181.

A. bone

B. blood-brain barrier

C. meninges

D. pia mater

E. dural sinuses

F. ventricles

G. choroid plexus

H. dura mater

I. central canal

J. arachnoid

K. subarachnoid

L. arachnoid villi

1. __H__   tough outermost layer of the meninges; means *hard mother*

2. __G__   cerebrospinal fluid is formed from these blood vessels and glial cells (ependyma) that line the ventricular walls

3. __B__   the astrocytes help to form this capillary structure, which prevents harmful substances in the blood from diffusing into the brain and spinal cord

4. __A__   cranium and vertebral column

5. __K__   cerebrospinal fluid circulates around the brain and spinal cord within this space

6. __E__   cavities that are filled with blood and help drain the cerebrospinal fluid

7. __F__   called the *lateral, third,* and *fourth*

8. __D__   the soft innermost layer of the meninges; means *soft mother*

9. __L__   fingerlike structures that project into the dural sinuses to allow drainage of the cerebrospinal fluid

10. __I__   hole in the center of the spinal cord through which cerebrospinal fluid flows from the ventricles of the brain to the lower end of the spinal cord

11. __J__   the middle layer of the meninges; means *spider* because the layer looks like a spiderweb

12. __C__   composed of the dura mater, arachnoid, and pia mater

13. __H__   meningeal layer that forms the tentorium

Student Name _____

ORDERING

Cerebrospinal Fluid

Directions. Trace the formation of cerebrospinal fluid from its formation across the choroid plexus in the lateral ventricles to its absorption into the cerebral veins. Use the words listed below. See text pp. 180-181.

third ventricle   arachnoid villi   dural sinuses

cerebral veins   central canal or foramina   choroid plexus (lateral ventricles)

fourth ventricle   subarachnoid space

1. choroid plexus of the lateral ventricles
2. _third ventricle_
3. _fourth ventricle_
4. _central canal/foramina_
5. _subarachnoid space_
6. _arachoid villi_
7. _dural sinus_
8. cerebral veins

PART II: PUTTING IT ALL TOGETHER

MULTIPLE CHOICE

Directions. Choose the correct answer.

1. A nerve impulse that originates in the precentral gyrus of the cerebrum
   a. allows one to see.
   b. helps you to analyze the meaning of speech.
   c. increases respiratory rate.
   d. causes skeletal muscle contraction and movement.

2. The medulla oblongata is called (the)
   a. *vital center* because it plays an important role in the control of respirations and cardiac function.
   b. emotional brain.
   c. primary somatosensory area because it receives information about breathing and heart rate.
   d. Broca's area because it controls motor speech.

3. Which of the following is most descriptive of multiple sclerosis?

   a. a disease in which the myelin sheath is gradually replaced by scar tissue
   b. a neuromuscular disorder caused by a deficiency of dopamine
   c. brain death due to cerebral hypoxia
   d. increased intracranial pressure that causes downward displacement (herniation) of the brain stem

4. The central sulcus, lateral fissure, and longitudinal fissure

   a. separate or divide cerebral lobes.
   b. are found within the spinal cord.
   c. are located only on the right side of the brain.
   d. separate the cerebrum from the cerebellum.

5. The frontal, parietal, occipital, and temporal lobes

   a. are cerebral structures.
   b. comprise the brain stem.
   c. are parts of the diencephalon.
   d. only perform sensory functions.

6. A deficiency of the neurotransmitter in the basal nuclei

   a. stimulates the CTZ and emetic center.
   b. causes a type of motor impairment called *Parkinson's disease*.
   c. causes demyelination and multiple sclerosis.
   d. causes cortical blindness.

7. A rapid influx of sodium (Na^+) into a neuron

   a. makes the inside of the neuron more negative than resting membrane potential.
   b. causes repolarization.
   c. causes depolarization.
   d. prevents the firing of an action potential.

8. What is the result of damage to Broca's area?

   a. paralysis of all the extremities
   b. respiratory depression
   c. blindness
   d. inability to speak

9. A staggering gait and imbalance are most descriptive of

   a. damage to the occipital lobe.
   b. impaired function of the medulla oblongata.
   c. cerebellar dysfunction.
   d. stimulation of the CTZ.

10. Repolarization of a neuron occurs in response to

    a. a rapid influx of sodium.
    b. a rapid efflux of potassium.
    c. an influx of K^+.
    d. an influx of calcium.

11. The medulla oblongata, pons, and midbrain are

    a. parts of the brain stem.
    b. cerebral lobes.
    c. dopamine-secreting nuclei.
    d. auditory association areas.

12. What happens at a synapse?

    a. saltatory conduction
    b. formation of cerebrospinal fluid
    c. chemical transmission of information
    d. synthesis of myelin sheath

13. The choroid plexus is most concerned with

    a. memory.
    b. formation of cerebrospinal fluid.
    c. the drainage of cerebrospinal fluid.
    d. the integrity of the blood-brain barrier.

14. Saltatory conduction refers to the

    a. flow of the cerebrospinal fluid.
    b. movement of the nerve impulse.
    c. pH of the cerebrospinal fluid.
    d. blood flow through the brain.

15. Which of the following is most descriptive of ganglia?

    a. cells of the blood-brain barrier
    b. clusters of ependymal cells
    c. clusters of cell bodies
    d. myelinated fibers

16. Damage to the right side of the brain, as in stroke, results in paralysis to the left side of the body. Which of the following words explains this occurrence?

    a. decussation
    b. synapse
    c. homunculus
    d. placticity

17. In which structure does the cerebrospinal fluid not circulate?

    a. subarachnoid space
    b. corpus callosum
    c. ventricles
    d. central canal

18. Which of the following is least descriptive of the auditory area?

    a. hearing
    b. temporal lobe
    c. precentral gyrus
    d. sensory

19. What is the usual cause of impaired mental functioning in older adults?

    a. loss of frontal lobe neurons
    b. deterioration of Broca's area
    c. demyelination of all neurons within the CNS
    d. age-related diseases such as atherosclerosis

20. Who acts like she is in another world?

    a. Dora Mater
    b. Di Encephalon
    c. Nerve Anna
    d. Hy P. O'Thalamus

CASE STUDY

T.O., a professional boxer, sustained a severe blow to his head in round 8. As he left his corner to begin the 9th round, he collapsed to the floor. He was rushed to the emergency room in an unconscious state and was diagnosed with a subdural hematoma. He was placed in semi-Fowler's position and given steroids and a diuretic. Holes were drilled in his skull to relieve the intracranial pressure.

1. Where was the clot located?

    a. within a cerebral ventricle
    b. within the central sulcus
    c. under the outer layer of meninges
    d. in the frontal lobe

2. Which of the following is true about the blood clot?

    a. It may continue to expand as water is pulled into the clot.
    b. It will probably dissolve on its own, but generally causes blindness.
    c. It will stop enlarging as soon as the bleeding stops; no treatment is necessary after the bleeding stops.
    d. All blood clots in the brain are lethal, with or without treatment.

3. What caused the loss of consciousness? The

    a. blood clot was pressing on the brain and was causing an elevation in intracranial pressure.
    b. hematoma was producing a brain-toxic substance.
    c. blood clot was blocking the formation of cerebrospinal fluid.
    d. hematoma caused a brain abscess, since a clot is an excellent place for pathogens to grow.

PART III: CHALLENGE YOURSELF!

GROUPS AND PUZZLE

1. Which group is incorrect?

    a. parts of a neuron: dendrites, cell body, axon
    b. types of nerve cells: neurons, neuroglia
    c. meninges: pia mater, arachnoid, dura mater
    d. parts of the brain stem: corpus callosum, pons, medulla oblongata

2. Which group is incorrect?

    a. parts of a neuron: dendrites, cell body, axon
    b. types of nerve cells: neurons, neuroglia
    c. types of glia: astrocytes, ependymal cells, oligodendrocytes, gyri
    d. lobes of the cerebrum: frontal, parietal, occipital, temporal

3. Which group is incorrect?

    a. lobes of the cerebrum: frontal, parietal, occipital, temporal
    b. parts of the brain stem: midbrain, occipital lobe, medulla oblongata
    c. parts of the diencephalon: thalamus, hypothalamus
    d. electrical events: depolarization, repolarization, action potential

PUZZLE

Hint: The Itsy Bitsy Spider... in the CNS

Directions. Perform the following functions on the Sequence of Words below. When all the functions have been performed, you are left with word(s) that are related to the hint. Record your answer below.

Functions: remove the following

1. hard mother
2. type of glial cell concerned with the formation of cerebrospinal fluid
3. soft mother
4. the names of the four ventricles
5. cerebrospinal fluid circulates within here
6. the hole in the spinal cord through which cerebrospinal fluid flows
7. the cluster of capillaries across which cerebrospinal fluid is formed
8. blood-filled space that drains cerebrospinal fluid
9. cerebral lobes (4)
10. parts (3) of the brainstem

Sequence of Words

PIAMATERPONSFRONTALEPENDYMAMEDULLAOBLONGATACHOROIDPLEXUSPARI
ETALDURAMATERLATERALARACHNOIDCENTRALCANALTEMPORALTHIRDOCCIPITA
LFOURTHSUBARACHNOIDSPACEMIDBRAINDURALSINUS

Answer: ARACHOID

Nervous System: Spinal Cord and Peripheral Nerves

Answer Key: Textbook page references are provided as a guide for answering these questions. A complete answer key was provided for your instructor.

Objectives

1. Describe the anatomy of the spinal cord and list its three functions.

2. List four components of the reflex arc.

3. List and describe the functions of the 12 pairs of cranial nerves.

4. Identify the classification of spinal nerves.

5. List the functions of the three major plexuses.

PART I: MASTERING THE BASICS

MATCHING

Nerve Tracts

Directions. In the spaces provided, indicate whether the following are sensory (S) or motor (M) structures or functions. See text pp. 187-189.

1. __M__ descending tracts

2. __S__ carries information for touch, pressure, and pain

3. __M__ corticospinal tract

4. __M__ pyramidal tract

5. __S__ ascending tracts

6. __M__ electrical signal arises in the precentral gyrus of the frontal lobe

7. __S__ carries information to the parietal lobe

8. __S__ first, second, and eighth cranial nerves

9. __M__ extrapyramidal tracts

10. __S__ spinothalamic tract

11. __S__ I feel pain in my little finger.

12. __M__ I'm wiggling my toes.

13. __S__ I'm cold.

14. __M__ I'm winking.

15. __S__ I'm hearing voices.

Student Name _____

MATCHING

Reflexes

Directions. Match the following terms to the most appropriate definition by writing the correct letter in the space provided. See text pp. 191-193.

A. Babinski reflex
B. Achilles tendon reflex
C. gag reflex
D. baroreceptor reflex
E. patellar tendon reflex
F. withdrawal reflex
G. pupillary reflex

1. _F_   a protective reflex; it quickly moves your finger away from a hot object

2. _E_   this reflex helps you maintain a standing posture; also called the *knee-jerk reflex*

3. _D_   this reflex helps your body maintain a normal blood pressure

4. _A_   this reflex is elicited by stroking the sole of the foot; plantar flexion and curling of the toes are normal responses in an adult

5. _G_   this reflex causes the pupils of the eyes to constrict (become smaller) in response to light

6. _B_   a stretch reflex; tapping this tendon in the heel normally causes plantar flexion of the foot; also called the *ankle-jerk reflex*

7. _C_   this reflex involves the glossopharyngeal nerve and helps prevent food and water from going down the wrong way

READ THE DIAGRAM

Reflex Arc

Directions. Referring to Figure 11-5 in the textbook, fill in the spaces with the correct numbers. Some numbers may be used more than once. See text p. 191.

1. _4_   result of the contraction of the quadriceps femoris

2. _1_   receptors in the thigh muscles are stimulated

3. _3_   motor neuron

4. _2_   sensory neuron

5. _2_   afferent neuron

6. _3_   efferent neuron

7. _4_   extension of the leg

8. _3_   information travels from the spinal cord to the muscle

9. _2_   information travels from receptors in the muscle to the spinal cord

MATCHING

Cranial Nerves

Directions. Match the following terms to the most appropriate definition by writing the correct letter in the space provided. Some terms may be used more than once. See text pp. 194-197.

A. olfactory

B. vestibulocochlear

C. vagus

D. accessory

E. optic

F. hypoglossal

G. oculomotor

H. trigeminal

I. facial

1. __B__ senses hearing and balance

2. __C__ the wanderer; it is widely distributed throughout the thoracic and abdominal cavities

3. __F__ helps control the movements of the tongue; cranial nerve XII

4. __D__ allows you to shrug your shoulders

5. __E__ damage to this nerve causes blindness

6. __A__ sense of smell

7. __H__ tic douloureux, a condition characterized by extreme facial and jaw pain, is caused by inflammation of this nerve; triggers include eating, shaving, and exposure to cold temperatures

8. __G__ a dilated and fixed pupil is caused by pressure on this nerve

9. __I__ inflammation of this nerve causes Bell's palsy, a paralysis of one side of the face

10. __G__ nerve that supplies most of the extrinsic eye muscles; primary function is the movement of the eyeballs

11. __E__ carries sensory information from the eyes to the occipital lobe of the brain

12. __G__ in addition to moving the eyeball, this nerve raises the eyelid and constricts the pupil of the eye

13. __A__ anosmia

14. __B__ cranial nerve VIII

15. __B__ ototoxicity

16. __G__ ptosis of the lids

17. __E__ cranial nerve II

18. __B__ vertigo

19. __I__ can't smile, wrinkle forehead, secrete tears, or close eyes (on the affected side)

20. __C__ cranial nerve X

Student Name _____

MATCHING

Spinal Nerves

Directions. Match the following terms to the most appropriate definition by writing the correct letter in the space provided. Some terms may be used more than once. See text pp. 197-201.

A. sciatic   D. pudendal   G. phrenic

B. axillary   E. femoral   H. plexus(es)

C. radial   F. cauda equina   I. common peroneal

1. __C__   wristdrop is caused by damage to this nerve

2. __B__   crutch palsy is caused by damage to this nerve

3. __G__   nerve that supplies the diaphragm, an important breathing muscle

4. __H__   spinal nerves are grouped and sorted here

5. __A__   this large nerve leaves or emerges from the distal end of the spinal cord and supplies the buttocks and posterior thighs

6. __H__   nerve groupings that are described as cervical, brachial, and lumbosacral nerves

7. __D__   deadening of this nerve assists in childbirth

8. __F__   group of nerves that emerge from the distal end of the spinal cord; horse's tail

9. __E__   innervates the inner thigh area

10. __I__   if damaged, causes footdrop

11. __A__   must administer an intramuscular (IM) injection in the upper outer quadrant of the buttocks in order to avoid injuring this nerve

12. __G__   severing this nerve requires the use of a ventilator

PART II: PUTTING IT ALL TOGETHER

MULTIPLE CHOICE

Directions. Choose the correct answer.

1. Which of the following is most descriptive of a descending tract?

    a. afferent
    b. sensory
    c. spinothalamic
    d. motor

2. Which of the following is most likely to experience ototoxicity?

    a. a furniture mover who strained his back
    b. a person who was diagnosed with a tumor involving the second cranial nerve
    c. a person who took an antibiotic drug that injured CN VIII
    d. a person with Bell's palsy

3. The pyramidal tract is

    a. the major motor tract that originates in the precentral gyrus.
    b. an ascending tract.
    c. a sensory tract.
    d. also called the *spinothalamic tract*.

4. A student nurse is instructed to administer an IM injection in the upper outer quadrant of the buttocks in order to

    a. prevent ototoxicity.
    b. minimize systemic effects of the drug.
    c. avoid penetration of the subarachnoid space.
    d. avoid injury to the sciatic nerve.

5. Which of the following is a function of the spinal cord?

    a. secretes hormones that regulate blood glucose
    b. is the seat of our emotions
    c. acts as an important reflex center
    d. secretes cerebrospinal fluid

6. Which of the following is least related to the others?

    a. pyramidal tract
    b. extrapyramidal tract
    c. spinothalamic tract
    d. corticospinal tract

7. What is the purpose of myelination?

    a. increases the speed of the nerve impulse
    b. prevents the release of neurotransmitter
    c. increases the phagocytic activity of the glia
    d. separates neurons from the surrounding glia

8. Which of the following is least descriptive of the vagus nerve?

    a. CN X
    b. distributed throughout the chest and abdomen
    c. an inflamed vagus nerve causes Bell's palsy
    d. affects the function of the digestive tract

9. Which of the following is a true statement?

    a. The olfactory nerve is a motor nerve.
    b. The second cranial nerve is a sensory nerve.
    c. The phrenic, sciatic, and axillary nerves are cranial nerves.
    d. The vagus nerve is confined to the cranium.

10. Which of the following is most descriptive of the cauda equina?

    a. spinal nerves that emerge from the tail-end of the spinal cord
    b. cells that secrete cerebrospinal fluid
    c. glial cells that form the blood-brain barrier
    d. meninges

11. Diagnostically, a needle is inserted between the third and fourth lumbar vertebrae into the subarachnoid space in order to

    a. relieve intracranial pressure from a closed head injury.
    b. obtain a sample of cerebrospinal fluid.
    c. stimulate myelination in the patient with multiple sclerosis.
    d. assess dopamine-secreting cells in the basal ganglia.

Student Name _____

12. These nerves supply voluntary skeletal muscles causing movement.

    a. somatic motor nerves
    b. vagus nerve
    c. parasympathetic nerves
    d. sympathetic nerves

13. A mixed nerve is one that

    a. only transmits information for pain.
    b. only transmits information that originates in the precentral gyrus.
    c. contains both sensory and motor fibers.
    d. only affects organs that are in the abdominal cavity.

14. Which involuntary response to a stimulus is accomplished by these four structures: receptor, sensory neuron, motor neuron, effector organ?

    a. action potential
    b. decussation
    c. reflex
    d. saltatory conduction

15. What is the effector organ in the knee-jerk or patellar tendon reflex?

    a. patella
    b. quadriceps femoris muscle
    c. spinal cord
    d. sole of the foot

16. Which of the following is least descriptive of the oculomotor nerve?

    a. CN III
    b. controls the movement of the eyeball
    c. increased intracranial pressure compresses this nerve and causes ptosis of the eyelid
    d. carries sensory information from the eye to the occipital lobe (vision)

17. Which of the following is a consequence of damage to the glossopharyngeal nerve?

    a. inability to shrug the shoulders and move the upper extremities
    b. blindness
    c. loss of the gag reflex and aspiration of food or water into the lungs
    d. loss of balance

18. The phrenic nerve

    a. is a cranial nerve.
    b. exits the spinal cord at the level of T12.
    c. innervates the major breathing muscle.
    d. is classified exclusively as ascending and sensory.

19. The first three cranial nerves

    a. are all sensory.
    b. innervate the eye.
    c. are all motor.
    d. are the olfactory, optic, and oculomotor nerves.

20. Who likes to have the sole of his foot stroked?

    a. Broca
    b. Cy Atica
    c. Achilles
    d. Babinksi

CASE STUDY

Jake and his friends were picnicking near a river. He dove into the river, hitting his head on a submerged rock. When he was pulled from the river by his friends, Jake was conscious but unable to move his body. There was no feeling in his upper or lower extremities. The paramedics stabilized his neck and spinal cord and transported him to the nearest trauma center. He had sustained a fracture at the C7 and C8 vertebrae.

1. Which of the following is indicated by the paralysis?

    a. The break was accompanied by hemorrhage and severe blood loss.
    b. An infection developed at the fracture site.
    c. The spinal cord had been severed.
    d. Severe brain damage had also occurred.

2. Which of the following words best describes Jake's loss of function?

    a. subdural hematoma
    b. increased intracranial pressure
    c. quadriplegia
    d. poliomyelitis

3. Which statement is true regarding Jake's long-term recovery?

    a. Complete recovery is likely within a 3-month period.
    b. He will regain all motor activity but will not regain any sensory function.
    c. He will require a ventilator to breathe and should regain full use of his upper and lower extremities within 3 months.
    d. It is unlikely that he will regain full use of either his upper or lower extremities.

4. Which statement best explains the reason for the above answer?

    a. Neurons within the CNS do not regenerate.
    b. The reticular activating system reacts to trauma by "closing down;" a deep coma ensues.
    c. Severe injury stops the formation of cerebrospinal fluid.
    d. Injured neurons regenerate but take several months to do so.

PART III: CHALLENGE YOURSELF!

GROUPS AND PUZZLE

1. Which group is incorrect?

    a. cranial nerves: olfactory, optic, oculomotor
    b. plexuses: cervical, brachial, lumbosacral
    c. states of paralysis: paralysis, quadriplegia, dermatome
    d. spinal nerves: phrenic, axillary, and sciatic

2. Which group is incorrect?

    a. states of paralysis: paraplegia, quadriplegia, hemiplegia
    b. nerve damage: crutch palsy, wristdrop, footdrop, Bell's palsy
    c. cranial nerves: oculomotor, phrenic, vagus, vestibulocochlear
    d. sensory nerves: olfactory, CN I, optic, CN VIII

Student Name _____

3. Which group is incorrect?

    a. spinal nerves: phrenic, axillary, sciatic
    b. reflexes: baroreceptor, withdrawal, pupillary, gag
    c. nerve damage: crutch palsy, wristdrop, footdrop, Bell's palsy
    d. motor nerves: descending, efferent, spinothalamic

PUZZLE

Hint: Cleopatra's Favorite Motor Tract

Directions. Perform the following functions on the Sequence of Words below. When all the functions have been performed, you are left with word(s) that are related to the hint. Record your answer below.

Functions: remove the following

1. five cranial nerves

2. innervates the diaphragm

3. three nerve plexuses

4. consequences of severing CNs II and VIII

5. nerve damaged with crutch palsy

6. nerves that carry information toward the CNS

7. nerves that carry information from the CNS toward the effector organs such as the muscles

8. mapping of the skin indicating specific innervation

9. nerve damaged in carpal tunnel syndrome

10. clinical effects of inflammation of CN VII

Sequence of Words

DERMATOMEDEAFNESSBRACHIALAXILLARYCERVICALVESTIBULOCOCHLEARPHRENICSE
NSORYPYRAMIDALBELLSPALSYOPTICMEDIANOCULOMOTORLUMBOSACRALVAGUSBLI
NDNESSOLFACTORYCORTICOSPINALMOTOR

Answer: PYRAMIDAL , CORTICOSPINAL

Autonomic Nervous System

Answer Key: Textbook page references are provided as a guide for answering these questions. A complete answer key was provided for your instructor.

Objectives

1. Describe the function of the autonomic nervous system.

2. Identify the two divisions of the autonomic nervous system.

3. State the anatomical and functional differences between the sympathetic and parasympathetic nervous systems.

4. Define cholinergic and adrenergic fibers.

5. Name the major neurotransmitters of the autonomic nervous system.

6. Name and locate the cholinergic and adrenergic receptors.

7. Explain the terms used to describe the effects of drugs on autonomic receptors.

MATCHING

Autonomic Nervous System

Directions. In the spaces provided, indicate whether the following describe sympathetic (S) or parasympathetic (P) nervous system effects. See text pp. 204-206.

1. __S__ thoracolumbar outflow
2. __P__ feed-and-breed
3. __S__ paravertebral ganglia
4. __S__ stressed-out and uptight
5. __P__ craniosacral outflow
6. __P__ paradoxical fear, "bradying down"
7. __S__ adrenergic
8. __S__ vasomotor tone
9. __S__ fight-or-flight

READ THE DIAGRAM

Directions. Refer to Figure 12-2 in the textbook and indicate if the statement is true (T) or false (F). See text p. 207.

1. __F__ the paravertebral ganglia are present in both the parasympathetic nervous system (PNS) and sympathetic nervous system (SNS)
2. __T__ the preganglionic fibers of the PNS and SNS are cholinergic
3. __F__ the postganglionic fibers of the PNS and SNS are cholinergic
4. __F__ the postganglionic fibers of the PNS and SNS are adrenergic
5. __T__ the preganglionic fibers of the SNS exit the spinal cord at the thoracolumbar region
6. __T__ the transmitter for the postganglionic fibers of the SNS is norepinephrine (NE)
7. __T__ the transmitter for the postganglionic fibers of the PNS is acetylcholine (ACh)
8. __T__ the preganglionic and postganglionic fibers associated with the craniosacral outflow are cholinergic
9. __T__ the transmitter of the preganglionic fibers of both the PNS and SNS is ACh
10. __T__ fibers colored green are cholinergic
11. __T__ fibers colored red are adrenergic
12. __F__ all autonomic fibers are colored red

Student Name _____

13. __T__ preganglionic fibers of the parasympathetic nervous system are longer than the preganglionic fibers of the sympathetic nervous system

14. __T__ drugs that block the effects of ACh affect both the sympathetic and parasympathetic nervous systems

15. __F__ drugs that block the effects of NE affect both the sympathetic and parasympathetic nervous
systems

READ THE DIAGRAM

Autonomic Receptors

*Directions. Refer to Figure 12-3 in the textbook and indicate if the statement is true (T) or false (F).
See text p. 210.*

1. __T__ the postganglionic receptors for the PNS are muscarinic

2. __F__ muscarinic receptors are activated by norepinephrine (NE)

3. __T__ α (alpha) and β (beta) receptors are activated by NE

4. __T__ the postganglionic receptors for the SNS are called α (alpha) and β (beta) receptors

5. __T__ fibers that are colored green secrete ACh as their transmitter

6. __T__ fiber that are colored red secrete NE as their transmitter

7. __F__ nicotinic receptors are found only in the autonomic nervous system

8. __T__ the transmitter of the preganglionic fibers of both the PNS and SNS activate nicotinic receptors

9. __T__ a drug that blocks muscarinic receptors diminishes the parasympathetic response

10. __T__ a drug that blocks alpha or beta receptors diminishes a sympathetic response

11. __T__ muscarinic and nicotinic receptors are cholinergic receptors

12. __T__ alpha and beta receptors are adrenergic receptors

13. __F__ cholinergic fibers are found only in the autonomic nervous system

14. __T__ a drug that affects the N_N receptors affects both the PNS and SNS

15. __T__ nicotinic receptors within the neuromuscular junction are activated by ACh

16. __T__ nicotinic receptors are located in both the PNS and SNS

17. __T__ a drug that blocks the N_M receptors within the neuromuscular junction causes skeletal
muscle paralysis

DRAW IT

Receptor Shapes and Fit

Directions. Refer to Figure 12-3 in the textbook and draw the following shapes.

1. Draw the shape of the muscarinic receptor. Draw the shape of ACh that fits into this receptor.

2. Draw the shape of the alpha or beta receptor. Draw the shape of the NE that fits into this receptor.

3. Draw the shape of the nicotinic N_M receptor. Draw the shape of the ACh the fits into the receptor.

MATCHING

Sympathetic or Parasympathetic Effects

Directions. Indicate if the following is a sympathetic effect (S) or a parasympathetic effect (P). See text pp. 209-212.

1. __S__ increased heart rate

2. __S__ dilation of the pupils of the eyes

3. __S__ dilation of the breathing passages

4. __P__ stimulation of urination

5. __S__ increased blood pressure

6. __S__ vasoconstriction

7. __P__ decreased heart rate

8. __S__ stronger heart muscle contraction

9. __P__ constriction of the pupil of the eye

10. __S__ increased perspiration

11. __S__ pounding heart and sweaty palms

12. __S__ anxiety and tremors

Student Name _____

PART II: PUTTING IT ALL TOGETHER

MULTIPLE CHOICE

Directions. Choose the correct answer.

1. Sympathetic and parasympathetic nerves

    a. are somatic motor neurons.
    b. supply the voluntary skeletal muscles.
    c. include the phrenic, sciatic, and brachial nerves.
    d. innervate the viscera.

2. Which of the following is least true of the sympathetic nervous system?

    a. fight-or-flight
    b. preganglionic fibers are cholinergic
    c. postganglionic fibers are adrenergic
    d. the postganglionic receptor is muscarinic

3. Which of the following is most descriptive of the parasympathetic nervous system?

    a. fight-or-flight
    b. preganglionic fibers are adrenergic
    c. postganglionic fibers are adrenergic
    d. the postganglionic receptor is muscarinic

4. Stimulation of the SNS causes the heart to beat stronger and faster. A drug that also causes the heart to beat stronger and faster is described as

    a. parasympatholytic.
    b. vagomimetic.
    c. sympathomimetic.
    d. sympatholytic.

5. Vasomotor tone is

    a. a vasoconstrictor effect caused by background firing of the sympathetic nerves.
    b. a vagally induced vasoconstriction.
    c. a response to activation of the muscarinic receptors on the blood vessels.
    d. caused by a beta adrenergic antagonist.

6. What is the clinical consequence of loss of vasomotor tone?

    a. urticaria and pruritus
    b. lethargy and jaundice
    c. severe decline in blood pressure and shock
    d. elevation in blood pressure and hemorrhage

7. Paravertebral ganglia

    a. contain beta adrenergic receptors that are activated by NE.
    b. are part of the craniosacral outflow.
    c. are located within the sympathetic nervous system.
    d. are located within the effector organs.

8. Which of the following is least descriptive of the thoracolumbar outflow?

    a. fight-or-flight
    b. muscarinic and nicotinic receptors
    c. sympathetic nervous system
    d. paravertebral ganglia

9. Alpha and beta adrenergic receptors are

    a. associated with the parasympathetic nervous system.
    b. associated with craniosacral outflow.
    c. located on the paravertebral ganglia.
    d. activated by norepinephrine.

10. The adrenal medulla secretes epinephrine and norepinephrine; the effects of the hormones are best described as

    a. vagolytic.
    b. sympathomimetic.
    c. parasympathomimetic.
    d. sympatholytic.

11. Which of the following fibers secretes norepinephrine (NE)?

    a. preganglionic sympathetic
    b. preganglionic parasympathetic
    c. postganglionic sympathetic
    d. postganglionic parasympathetic

12. Which of the following is least descriptive of monoamine oxidase (MAO)?

    a. enzyme that degrades NE
    b. found within all cholinergic fibers
    c. associated with sympathetic activity
    d. associated with adrenergic fibers

13. A β_1 adrenergic agonist

    a. increases heart rate.
    b. causes the release of acetylcholine.
    c. blocks the effects of NE at its receptor site.
    d. lowers blood pressure.

14. Atropine is classified as a muscarinic blocker and therefore is

    a. parasympathomimetic.
    b. sympatholytic.
    c. vagolytic.
    d. sympathomimetic.

15. Muscarinic receptors are located on

    a. the paravertebral ganglia.
    b. the effector organs: postganglionic parasympathetic.
    c. the effector organs: postganglionic sympathetic.
    d. all autonomic ganglia.

16. Sympathetic nervous system stimulation causes vasoconstriction of the blood vessels, thereby elevating blood pressure. Which of the following drugs lowers blood pressure?

    a. vagolytic
    b. sympathomimetic
    c. α_1 adrenergic blocker
    d. β_2 adrenergic agonist

17. Sympathetic nervous system stimulation causes relaxation of the breathing passages (i.e., bronchodilation). Which of the following drugs achieves this effect?

    a. β_2 adrenergic agonist
    b. α_1 blocker
    c. muscarinic antagonist
    d. vagomimetic

18. A patient received an antimuscarinic drug (atropine) preoperatively. What drug-related postoperative consequence is he likely to experience?

    a. slow heart rate
    b. inability to urinate
    c. excess salivation
    d. pinpoint pupils

CASE STUDY

A patient has had a heart attack and is experiencing a very slow heart rate because of intense parasympathetic discharge.

1. Which of the following drugs will increase his heart rate?

    a. vagolytic
    b. α_1 agonist
    c. β_1 adrenergic antagonist
    d. muscarinic agonist

2. Restate the answer in question #1.

    a. sympatholytic
    b. parasympatholytic
    c. parasympathomimetic
    d. muscarinic agonist

3. What would happen if a muscarinic agonist were administered?

    a. heart rate would increase to normal
    b. heart rate would become too rapid
    c. his breathing would cease
    d. heart rate would decrease further

Student Name _____

PART III: CHALLENGE YOURSELF!

GROUPS AND PUZZLE

1. Indicate which group is incorrect.

   a. Adrenergic receptors: alpha and beta
   b. Cholinergic receptors: nicotinic and muscarinic
   c. Sympathetic terms: paravertebral ganglia, fight-or-flight, craniosacral outflow
   d. Parasympathetic terms: craniosacral outflow, feed-and-breed, muscarinic, and nicotinic

2. Indicate which group is incorrect.

   a. Adrenergic receptors: alpha and beta
   b. Cholinergic receptors: nicotinic, muscarinic, and dopaminergic
   c. Sympathetic terms: paravertebral ganglia, fight-or-flight, thoracolumbar outflow
   d. Parasympathetic terms: craniosacral outflow, feed-and-breed, muscarinic, and nicotinic

PUZZLE

Hint: "An Autonomic Blood Pressure Event"

Directions. Perform the following functions on the Sequence of Words below. When all the functions have been performed, you are left with word(s) that are related to the hint. Record your answer below.

Functions: remove the following

1. neurotransmitter for cholinergic fibers

2. an "outflow" name for the sympathetic nervous system

3. name of the sympathetic ganglia that run parallel to the spinal cord

4. neurotransmitter for adrenergic fibers

5. name of a cholinergic receptor

6. an "outflow" name for the parasympathetic nervous system

7. name of the parasympathetic nerve that innervates the heart

8. name of two adrenergic receptors

9. name of a drug that is classified as a beta$_1$ adrenergic blocker

10. name of a drug that is classified as a muscarinic blocker (anticholinergic)

Sequence of Words

PARAVERTEBRALALPHAPROPRANOLOLBETANOREPINEPHRINEVAGUSACETYLCHOLIN
EBARORECEPTORREFLEXMUSCARINICATROPINETHORACOLUMBARCRANIOSACRAL

Answer: _BARORECEPTOR REFLEX_

14

Endocrine System

Answer Key: Textbook page references are provided as a guide for answering these questions. A complete answer key was provided for your instructor.

Objectives

1. List the functions of the endocrine system.

2. Define hormone.

3. Explain negative feedback control as a regulator for hormone levels.

4. Describe the relationship of the hypothalamus to the pituitary gland.

5. Describe the location, hormones, and regulation of the pituitary gland.

6. Identify the major endocrine glands and their hormones.

7. Explain the effects of hyposecretion and hypersecretion of the major endocrine glands.

PART I: MASTERING THE BASICS

MATCHING

Hormone Action

Directions. Match the following terms to the most appropriate definition by writing the correct letter in the space provided. Some terms may be used more than once. See text pp. 239-243.

A. target tissue (organ)   D. endocrine glands   G. biorhythm(s)

B. receptor   E. exocrine glands   H. tropic hormones

C. hormones   F. negative feedback control   I. second chemical messenger

1. _____   type of glands that secrete hormones; called *ductless glands*

2. _____   type of glands that secrete into ducts; examples include sweat glands, sebaceous glands, and glands that secrete digestive enzymes

3. _____   hormones that are "aimed at" a target

4. _____   describes this pattern of hormone secretion: cortisol secretion is highest in the morning (8 AM) and lowest in the evening (midnight)

5. _____   endocrine secretions that are classified as proteins, protein-like substances, or steroids

6. _____   describes a specific tissue or organ to which a hormone binds

7. _____   describes, for example, this sequence of events: corticotropin-releasing hormone (CRH) stimulates the release of adrenocorticotropic hormone (ACTH), which in turn stimulates the secretion of cortisol; as the blood level of cortisol increases, it shuts off the further secretion of ACTH and CRH

8. _____   an example is a circadian rhythm

9. _____   jet lag and night-shift work alter this pattern of hormone secretion

10. _____   cAMP

11. _____   hormones bind to these special areas in the cell or on the surface of the cell membrane of the target tissue

12. _____   an example is the menstrual cycle

Student Name _____

MATCHING

Glands

Directions. Match the following terms to the most appropriate definition by writing the correct letter in the space provided. Some terms may be used more than once. See text pp. 243-258.

A. thyroid gland

B. anterior pituitary gland

C. posterior pituitary gland

D. hypothalamus

E. pancreas

F. pineal gland

G. parathyroid glands

H. adrenal cortex

I. adrenal medulla

J. ovaries

K. testes

L. thymus gland

1. _____   beta and alpha cells of the islets of Langerhans

2. _____   gonads that secrete estrogen and progesterone

3. _____   secretes T_3, T_4, and calcitonin

4. _____   secretes releasing hormones

5. _____   secretes antidiuretic hormone (ADH) and oxytocin

6. _____   called the *neurohypophysis*

7. _____   the hypothalamus and this gland are parts of the hypothalamic-hypophyseal portal system

8. _____   called the *adenohypophysis*

9. _____   secretes tropic hormones such as thyroid-stimulating hormone (TSH), ACTH, growth hormone (somatotropic hormone), and the gonadotropins

10. _____   secretes the catecholamines, epinephrine, and norepinephrine

11. _____   secretes the steroids: glucocorticoids, mineralocorticoids, and androgens

12. _____   target gland for ACTH

13. _____   low plasma levels of calcium stimulate these glands to secrete PTH

14. _____   secretes insulin and glucagon

15. _____   uses iodine to synthesize its hormones

16. _____   target gland of TSH

17. _____   secretions of this gland contribute to the fight-or-flight response

18. _____   the gonad that secretes testosterone

19. _____   this gland is associated with these words: *isthmus, follicular cells, colloid,* and *iodine*

20. _____   this gland plays an important role in immunity and involutes, or shrinks, after puberty

21. _____   secretes the hormones that are concerned with sugar, salt, and sex

22. _____   a cone-shaped gland located in the brain; it secretes melatonin and is called the *biologic clock*

23. _____   gland that enlarges as a goiter

24. _____   glands that are sometimes embedded within the thyroid gland; removal causes hypocalcemic tetany

MATCHING

Hormones

Directions. Match the following terms to the most appropriate definition by writing the correct letter in the space provided. Some terms may be used more than once. See text pp. 243-258.

A. catecholamines

B. steroids

C. insulin

D. glucagon

E. parathyroid hormone

F. growth hormone

G. gonadotropins

H. T_3 and T_4

I. calcitonin

J. ACTH

K. releasing hormones

L. melanocyte-stimulating hormone (MSH)

M. ADH

N. oxytocin

O. prolactin

1. _____ also called *somatotropic hormone,* this anterior pituitary hormone stimulates the growth of the musculoskeletal system

2. _____ the only hormone that lowers blood glucose

3. _____ cortisol, aldosterone, and testosterone

4. _____ epinephrine and norepinephrine; sympathomimetic hormones

5. _____ pancreatic hormone that increases blood glucose

6. _____ hormone that acts on three target organs (bone, kidneys, and intestine) to increase the blood levels of calcium

7. _____ stimulates the melanocytes to secrete a pigment that tans or darkens skin

8. _____ TSH stimulates the thyroid gland to release these hormones

9. _____ include follicle-stimulating hormone (FSH) and luteinizing hormone (LH)

10. _____ stimulates the breasts to make milk; also called *lactogenic hormone*

11. _____ posterior pituitary hormone that initiates labor

12. _____ parafollicular cells, thyroid gland, stimulates osteoblastic activity

13. _____ iodine-containing hormones that regulate BMR

14. _____ posterior pituitary hormone that stimulates the kidneys to reabsorb water

15. _____ hypothalamic hormones that control the hormonal secretion of the anterior pituitary gland

16. _____ tropic hormone that stimulates the adrenal cortex to secrete cortisol

17. _____ the stimulus for its release is an increasing blood glucose level

18. _____ posterior pituitary hormone that is secreted in response to a low blood volume and concentrated blood, as occurs in dehydration

19. _____ stimulates osteoclastic activity

20. _____ posterior pituitary hormone that is involved in the release of milk from the breast (the milk let-down reflex)

21. _____ also called *vasopressin*

22. _____ a decrease in plasma calcium is the stimulus for its release

Student Name _____

READ THE DIAGRAM

Directions. Referring to the diagram, fill in the spaces with the correct numbers. Some numbers may be used more than once. See text p. 240.

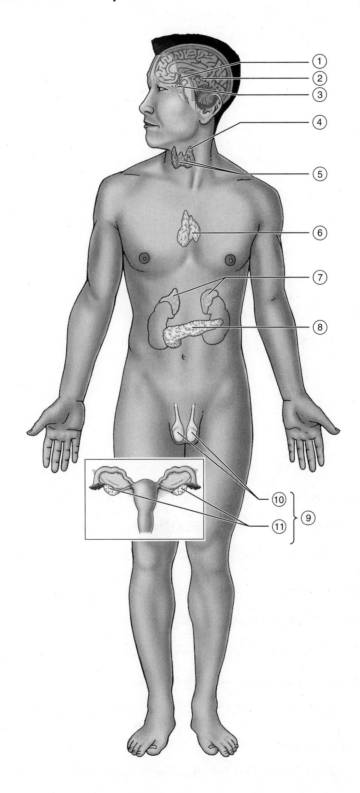

1. _____ gland that contains the alpha and beta cells of the islets of Langerhans

2. _____ gonads that secrete estrogen and progesterone

3. _____ a deficiency of this gland causes diabetes insipidus

4. _____ secretes T$_3$ and T$_4$ and calcitonin

5. _____ secretes releasing hormones

6. _____ secretes ADH and oxytocin

7. _____ a deficiency of this gland causes cretinism and myxedema

8. _____ a deficiency of this gland causes hypocalcemic tetany

9. _____ called the *hypophysis*

10. _____ the hypothalamus and this gland compose the hypothalamic-hypophyseal portal system

11. _____ secretes tropic hormones such as ACTH, TSH, growth hormone, and gonadotropins

12. _____ secretes the catecholamines, epinephrine, and norepinephrine

13. _____ secretes the steroids: glucocorticoids, mineralocorticoids, and androgens

14. _____ target gland for ACTH

15. _____ target gland for TSH

16. _____ secretes insulin and glucagon

17. _____ target gland (female) for FSH and LH

18. _____ target gland (male) for gonadotropins

19. _____ a low plasma level of calcium stimulates these glands to secrete PTH

20. _____ a high plasma level of calcium stimulates this gland to secrete calcitonin

21. _____ secretion of this gland contributes to the fight-or-flight response

22. _____ gland that secretes cortisol, aldosterone, and testosterone

23. _____ hypersecretion of this gland causes Cushing's syndrome

24. _____ hypersecretion of this gland causes Graves' disease

25. _____ hypersecretion of this gland is associated with exophthalmos

26. _____ gonad that secretes testosterone

27. _____ gland that utilizes iodine to synthesize its hormones

28. _____ gland that plays an important role in immunity and involutes, or shrinks, after puberty

Student Name _____

29. _____ secretes hormones concerned with sugar, salt, and sex

30. _____ a cone-shaped gland located in the brain; it is called the *biologic clock*

31. _____ gland that secretes the hormone that lowers blood glucose

32. _____ gland that secretes FSH and LH

33. _____ hormone that secretes lactogenic hormone

34. _____ gland that is the target gland for the releasing hormones

35. _____ gland that can develop a goiter

36. _____ gland that controls basal metabolic rate

37. _____ this gland secretes a hormone that promotes labor

38. _____ hypersecretion of this gland can cause giantism (childhood) or acromegaly (adult)

39. _____ hyposecretion of this gland causes Addison's disease

40. _____ gland that secretes both steroids and catecholamines

41. _____ refers to the male and female gonads

COLORING

Directions. Color the appropriate areas on the illustration on p. 155 as indicated below.

1. Color the pituitary gland ***red***.

2. Color the gland that secretes insulin and glucagon ***blue***.

3. Color the gland that secretes T_3 and T_4 ***yellow***.

4. Color the target gland of FSH and LH ***purple***.

5. Color the suprarenal glands ***pink***.

6. Color the parathyroid glands ***black***.

7. Color the thymus gland ***orange***.

MATCHING

Endocrine Disorders

Directions. Match the following terms to the most appropriate definition by writing the correct letter in the space provided. Some terms may be used more than once. See text pp. 243-258.

A. diabetes mellitus

B. Addison's disease

C. Cushing's syndrome

D. goiter

E. exophthalmos

F. Graves' disease

G. diabetes insipidus

H. pheochromocytoma

I. myxedema

J. tetany

K. acromegaly

L. giantism

M. dwarfism

N. cretinism

1. _____   this results from an iodine-deficient diet, which causes a hyperplasia or overgrowth of the thyroid gland

2. _____   results from a deficiency of insulin; the person becomes hyperglycemic and glucosuric

3. _____   condition that is due to a deficiency of adrenal cortical steroids

4. _____   results from a deficiency of ADH that causes the person to urinate up to 25 liters of pale urine per day

5. _____   condition that is treated with replacement doses of insulin

6. _____   the adult form of hypothyroidism that is treated with thyroid hormone

7. _____   antithyroid drugs and surgery are used to treat this form of hyperthyroidism

8. _____   an infant born with a deficiency of thyroid hormones develops this condition, characterized by a severe delay in both physical and mental development

9. _____   a deficiency of parathyroid hormone causes this life-threatening hypocalcemic condition

10. _____   condition that is caused by hypersecretion of growth hormone in an adult (after the fusion of the epiphyseal discs)

11. _____   condition that is caused by a hypersecretion of somatotropic hormone in a child

12. _____   condition that is caused by hyposecretion of somatotropic hormone in a child

13. _____   condition that results from a tumor of the adrenal medulla, which causes a very high (and dangerous) blood pressure

14. _____   describes the bulging or protruding eyes that characterize hyperthyroidism

15. _____   a person who takes high doses of steroids over an extended period of time will develop this group of signs and symptoms

16. _____   if untreated, this deficiency disease will progress to adrenal shock

17. _____   if untreated, this condition progresses to ketoacidosis

18. _____   characterized by sustained muscle contraction and an inability to ventilate (breathe)

19. _____   requires replacement doses of steroids, especially mineralocorticoid

20. _____   requires replacement doses of T_3 and T_4

TELL A STORY

Ms. Chvostek's Face Is A-Twitching

Directions. Use these words to complete the story. See text pp. 248-251.

(+) Chvostek's sign	osteoclastic activity	carpal spasm
PTH	(+) Trousseau's sign	parathyroid
kidney	laryngospasm	intestine
tetany		

Plasma levels of Ca^{2+} are regulated very tightly. As plasma Ca^{2+} decreases, the hormone _____ is secreted by the _____ glands. This hormone stimulates the _____ to reabsorb Ca^{2+} from the urine and the _____ to increase the absorption of dietary Ca^{2+}. Most importantly, the hormone stimulates _____; this action causes the Ca^{2+} to leave the bone and enter the plasma, thereby elevating plasma Ca^{2+}. So why is Ms. Chvostek's face a-twitching? Ms. Chvostek had her parathyroid glands surgically removed by accident (during a thyroidectomy). She subsequently developed hypocalcemia; this condition manifests itself clinically as _____ (a sustained muscle contraction). Two "muscle" signs of hypocalcemic tetany are _____ and _____. The Ca^{2+} imbalance also increases the nerve irritability, manifested clinically as _____ and _____.

PART II: PUTTING IT ALL TOGETHER

MULTIPLE CHOICE

Directions. Choose the correct answer.

1. Which of the following is least related to an endocrine gland?
   a. secretes hormones
   b. they are ductless glands
   c. secretions are transported by the blood
   d. all hormones are steroids

2. The adenohypophysis
   a. secretes only steroids.
   b. is controlled by the hypothalamus.
   c. is controlled by the posterior pituitary gland.
   d. requires iodine for the synthesis of TSH.

3. Complete this series: CRH → ACTH →
   a. T_3 and T_4
   b. cortisol
   c. insulin
   d. ADH

4. Complete this series: TRH → TSH →
   a. T_3 and T_4
   b. cortisol
   c. insulin
   d. ADH

5. Which of the following is true of insulin?
   a. secreted by the posterior pituitary gland
   b. a deficiency causes diabetes insipidus
   c. secreted in response to decreased blood glucose
   d. helps regulate blood glucose

6. Which of the following is not true of glucagon?
   a. lowers blood glucose
   b. synthesized by the pancreas
   c. synthesized by the islets of Langerhans
   d. opposes the action of insulin

7. Which of the following statements is true about ACTH?

    a. is a releasing hormone
    b. is secreted by the hypothalamus
    c. stimulates the adrenal cortex to secrete cortisol
    d. stimulates the adrenal medulla, initiating the fight-or-flight response

8. Which of the following is most related to FSH and LH?

    a. secreted by the pancreas
    b. are neurohypophyseal hormones
    c. regulate blood glucose
    d. tropic hormones that are aimed at the ovaries and testes

9. The ketoacidosis of diabetes mellitus is

    a. due to hyperglycemia.
    b. a consequence of glucosuria.
    c. due to the rapid and incomplete breakdown of fatty acids.
    d. due to an insulin-induced gluconeogenesis.

10. Hyperglycemia, glucosuria, and ketoacidosis are caused by

    a. excess secretion of ACTH by the anterior pituitary gland.
    b. a deficiency of ADH.
    c. a deficiency of insulin.
    d. outpouring of catecholamines by the adrenal medulla.

11. What characteristic is shared by both insulin and glucagon? Both

    a. are steroids.
    b. raise blood glucose.
    c. lower blood glucose.
    d. are secreted by the pancreas.

12. ACTH, TSH, and prolactin

    a. are secreted by the pancreas.
    b. are releasing hormones.
    c. stimulate the adrenal cortex to secrete cortisol.
    d. are synthesized by the adenohypophysis.

13. Which of the following is most related to the adrenal cortex?

    a. is the target gland of ACTH.
    b. regulates calcium homeostasis.
    c. secretes PTH.
    d. is imbedded within the thyroid gland.

14. BMR, iodine, myxedema, and Graves' disease are all

    a. concerned with T_3 and T_4.
    b. concerned with the regulation of plasma calcium.
    c. characterized by a low blood volume state.
    d. concerned with adenohypophyseal secretions.

15. Which statement is true about ADH?

    a. It is secreted by the anterior pituitary gland.
    b. It regulates blood volume.
    c. A deficiency causes hypervolemia.
    d. A deficiency causes oliguria (a decrease in urine excretion).

16. A deficiency of aldosterone

    a. causes a decrease in blood volume.
    b. causes diabetes insipidus.
    c. causes hyperglycemia, hypernatremia, and hyperkalemia.
    d. is called *Cushing's syndrome*.

17. Aldosterone

    a. stimulates the reabsorption of potassium by the kidney.
    b. causes the excretion of sodium in the urine.
    c. excretes water causing an increase in the output of urine.
    d. stimulates the reabsorption of sodium and water by the kidney.

18. PTH

    a. stimulates osteoclastic activity.
    b. lowers plasma calcium.
    c. elevates blood glucose.
    d. requires iodine for the synthesis of its hormones.

19. Which of the following statements is true regarding the aging process and the endocrine system?

    a. With aging, most glands decrease their hormonal secretion, resulting in severe clinical disorders such as diabetes mellitus and Addison's disease.
    b. Pheochromocytoma is the result of the normal aging process.
    c. Although most glands decrease their hormonal secretions, normal aging does not cause deficiency states.
    d. Most older adults suffer from osteoporosis and tetany.

Student Name _____

CASE STUDY

J.C., a 17-year-old high school senior, is a star football player and has just been awarded an athletic scholarship to college. About 8 months ago, he began using anabolic steroids to improve his athletic performance.

1. The steroids most resemble the secretions of which gland?

    a. pancreas
    b. adrenal medulla
    c. posterior pituitary gland
    d. adrenal cortex

2. What steroid-induced effect was J.C. expecting?

    a. increased muscle mass (bulking up) and strength
    b. decreased appetite
    c. decreased red blood cell production
    d. increased sex drive

PART III: CHALLENGE YOURSELF!

GROUPS AND PUZZLE

1. Which group is incorrect?

    a. hormones of the anterior pituitary gland: ACTH, prolactin, TSH, growth hormone, insulin
    b. hormones of the posterior pituitary gland: ADH, oxytocin
    c. steroids: cortisol, aldosterone, testosterone
    d. secretions of the gonads: estrogen, progesterone, testosterone

2. Which group is incorrect?

    a. hormones of the posterior pituitary gland: ADH, oxytocin
    b. steroids: cortisol, aldosterone, testosterone, estrogen
    c. secretions of the gonads: estrogen, progesterone, testosterone
    d. hormones secreted by the thyroid gland: T_3, T_4, PTH

3. Which group is incorrect?

    a. hormones of the anterior pituitary gland: ACTH, prolactin, TSH, growth hormone
    b. steroids: cortisol, aldosterone, testosterone
    c. secretions of the gonads: estrogen, progesterone, testosterone
    d. hormones secreted by the thyroid gland: TSH, T_3, T_4

PUZZLE

Hint: 'Roid Rage

Directions. Perform the following functions on the Sequence of Words below. When all the functions have been performed, you are left with word(s) that are related to the hint. Record your answer below.

Functions: remove the following

1. three classifications of adrenal steroids

2. the salt-retaining mineralocorticoid

3. two adrenal medullary catecholamines

4. a group of symptoms that are caused by excess secretion of the adrenal cortex

5. the condition caused by a chronic hypofunction of the adrenal cortex

6. the cation that is eliminated in the urine in response to aldosterone

7. the cation that is reabsorbed from the urine in response to aldosterone

8. the rounded face and supraclavicular fat pad caused by excess cortisol

9. disorder caused by excess secretion of the adrenal medulla (catecholamines)

10. ACTH stimulates the adrenal cortical secretion of this hormone

Sequence of Words

SODIUMMOONFACEMINERALOCORTICOIDCUSHINGSSYNDROMEPHEOCHROMOCYTOM
ACORTISOLEPINEPHRINEDRUG-INDUCEDAGGRESSIONGLUCOCORTICOIDBUFFALOHU
MPNOREPINEPHRINEADDISONSDISEASEALDOSTERONEANDROGENPOTASSIUM

Answer: _____

15

Blood

Answer Key: Textbook page references are provided as a guide for answering these questions. A complete answer key was provided for your instructor.

Objectives

1. Describe three functions of blood.

2. Describe the composition of blood.

3. Describe the three types of blood cells: erythrocytes, leukocytes, and thrombocytes.

4. Explain the formation of blood cells.

5. Explain the breakdown of red blood cells and the formation of bilirubin.

6. Identify the steps of hemostasis.

7. Describe the four blood types.

8. Describe the Rh factor.

PART I: MASTERING THE BASICS

MATCHING

Blood and Blood Tests

Directions. Match the following terms to the most appropriate definition by writing the correct letter in the space provided. Some terms may be used more than once. See text pp. 263-273.

A. plasma

B. hematopoiesis

C. hematocrit

D. hemoglobin

E. thrombocytes

F. leukocytes

G. bone marrow biopsy

H. erythrocytes

I. differential count

J. intrinsic factor

K. erythropoietin

L. hematology

M. bone marrow

N. blast cell

1. _____ white blood cells

2. _____ blood test that indicates the percentage of blood cells in a sample of blood

3. _____ component of the red blood cell to which the oxygen is attached

4. _____ protein secreted by the stomach that is necessary for the absorption of vitamin B_{12}

5. _____ red blood cells

6. _____ process of blood cell production

7. _____ blood test that indicates the percentage of each type of white blood cell in a sample of blood

8. _____ platelets

9. _____ hormone that stimulates the production of red blood cells

10. _____ liquid portion of the blood

11. _____ a sample of developing blood cells is withdrawn from the sternum or iliac crest; this procedure can detect abnormal blood cells

12. _____ part of the blood that contains the plasma proteins

13. _____ an immature cell

14. _____ tissue that makes blood cells

15. _____ tissue that is impaired in myelosuppression

16. _____ the study of blood

Student Name _____

READ THE DIAGRAM

Directions. Referring to Figure 15-2 in the textbook, fill in the blanks with the number of the column described by the statements below. See text p. 265.

1. _____ the maturation of the granulocytes
2. _____ the maturation of the oxygen-carrying blood cells
3. _____ the maturation of the cells that play a role in hemostasis
4. _____, _____, and _____ the maturation of the leukocytes
5. _____ the maturation of a myeloblast into a highly phagocytic cell
6. _____ the fragmentation of the megakaryocyte into the thrombocyte
7. _____ depression of the cells in this column causes granulocytopenia and infection
8. _____ depression of the cells in this column causes thrombocytopenia and bleeding
9. _____ the reticulocyte is an immature cell
10. _____ depression of this column causes anemia

MATCHING

Red Blood Cells, White Blood Cells, and Platelets

Directions. Indicate whether the following are most related to the red blood cell (RBC), white blood cell (WBC), or platelet (P) by writing the correct letter(s) in the space provided. See text pp. 265-279.

1. _____ small, highly phagocytic granulocyte
2. _____ antigens A and B
3. _____ delivers oxygen to the cells in the body
4. _____ a deficiency causes petechiae formation and bleeding
5. _____ the life span is about 120 days
6. _____ breaks down into protein, bilirubin, and iron
7. _____ includes lymphocytes and monocytes
8. _____ includes neutrophils, basophils, and eosinophils
9. _____ is filled primarily with hemoglobin
10. _____ the immature cell is the reticulocyte
11. _____ derived from the megakaryocyte
12. _____ is concerned primarily with phagocytosis
13. _____ is composed of granulocytes and agranulocytes
14. _____ leukocytosis and leukopenia
15. _____ characterized by diapedesis and chemotaxis
16. _____ is decreased in anemia
17. _____ primarily concerned with hemostasis
18. _____ synthesized in response to erythropoietin

19. _____ thrombocytopenia and bleeding

20. _____ granulocytopenia and infection

21. _____ contributes to the formation of pus

22. _____ the Rh factor

23. _____ its rapid breakdown causes jaundice

24. _____ the "culprit" in anemia

25. _____ plasma levels are monitored through changes in the hematocrit

26. _____ stickiness and plug

27. _____ involved in a hemolytic blood transfusion reaction

28. _____ intrinsic and extrinsic factors are necessary for its synthesis

29. _____ requires iron for its synthesis and function

30. _____ "shift-to-the-left"

31. _____ its rapid breakdown causes hyperbilirubinemia

TELL A STORY

Polly Cythemia and Her Oxygen

Directions. Complete the story by using the words below. Some words may be used more than once. See text pp. 267-268.

polycythemia	oxygen	kidneys
erythropoietin	anemia	red blood cells
hypoxic	bone marrow	myelosuppression

An older adult patient with emphysema was chronically hypoxic and developed an elevated hematocrit. Why, you ask? In response to the low tissue levels of oxygen, the _____ secrete the hormone _____. This hormone travels via the blood to the _____, where it stimulates the formation of _____. The increased amount of hemoglobin delivers more _____ to the tissues. Chronic hypoxia, therefore, causes a secondary _____ and an increase in hematocrit. There are other clinical conditions that involve erythropoietin. Patients in renal failure develop _____ (a deficiency of red blood cells) because of the lack of erythropoietin. Patients receiving cancer chemotherapy receive Epoetin (an erythropoietin-like drug) because of a chemotherapy-induced _____ and _____ (decreased red blood cells). Finally, athletes who train "at altitude" become mildly _____, and therefore secrete erythropoietin; in response they too develop a secondary _____.

Student Name _____

READ THE DIAGRAM

Breakdown of the Red Blood Cell

Directions. Referring to the illustration (Figure 15-6 in the textbook), indicate the breakdown products of the red blood cell by writing the correct numbers in the blanks. See text p. 269.

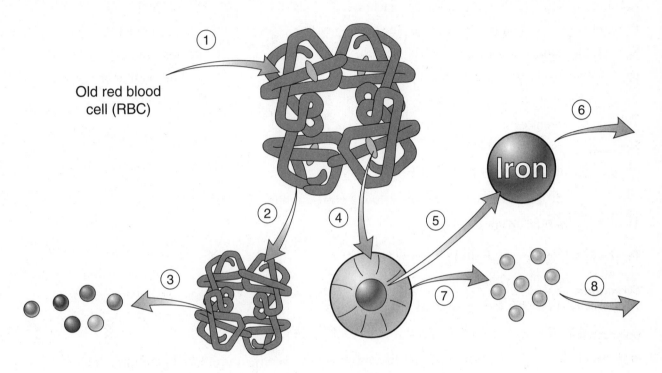

1. _____, _____ the consequences of hemoglobin degradation

2. _____, _____ the consequences of heme degradation

3. _____ hemoglobin leaves the aged erythrocyte

4. _____ the excretory route for bilirubin

5. _____ the heme is degraded to a ferrous element

6. _____ What happens to globin?

7. _____ What happens to the Fe?

MATCHING

Hemostasis

Directions. Match the following terms to the most appropriate definition by writing the correct letter in the space provided. See text pp. 273-276.

A. thrombus

B. prothrombin activator

C. fibrin threads

D. embolus

E. hemostasis

F. calcium

G. thrombin

H. heparin

I. Coumadin

J. fibrinolysis

K. plasmin

L. thrombolytics

M. hemolysis

N. coagulation process

O. platelets

1. _____ stoppage of bleeding

2. _____ a blood clot

3. _____ drug that decreases the formation of prothrombin in the liver

4. _____ a traveling or moving blood clot

5. _____ causes hypoprothrombinemia

6. _____ stickiness and plug

7. _____ its effects are reversed by vitamin K

8. _____ enzyme that converts prothrombin to thrombin

9. _____ element necessary for prothrombin activator to convert prothrombin to thrombin

10. _____ enzyme that dissolves clots

11. _____ prolongs the prothrombin time

12. _____ drugs that are called *clot busters*

13. _____ protein strands that actually form the blood clot

14. _____ derived from the megakaryocyte

15. _____ an anticoagulant that removes thrombin from the clotting process

16. _____ bursting of red blood cells

17. _____ enzyme that activates fibrinogen to fibrin

18. _____ thrombocytes

19. _____ refers to the series of reactions that results in the formation of a blood clot

20. _____ the target of aspirin

21. _____ process that dissolves a blood clot

TELL A STORY

Got a Clot

Directions. Complete the story by using the words below. See text pp. 273-276.

fibrinogen   prothrombin time   heparin

prothrombin   antithrombin   thrombin

Coumadin   hypoprothrombinemia

Mr. Flea Bitis, was admitted to the hospital with a diagnosis of deep vein thrombosis (DVT), a life-threatening condition associated with clot formation in the veins of the legs. He was given the drug _____ by intravenous (IV) infusion. This anticoagulant is an _____ agent. The drug-induced removal of _____ prevents the conversion of fibrinogen to fibrin threads (the clot). On the following day, he was also given _____, an oral anticoagulant. This anticoagulant works by preventing the hepatic utilization of vitamin K in the synthesis of _____. The goal of oral anticoagulant therapy is to cause _____; confirmed by a prolonged _____, a lab test used to monitor therapy. The intravenous anticoagulant was discontinued within the first week; however, the oral anticoagulant was continued for several months until the thrombotic condition was resolved.

MATCHING

Blood Types

Directions. Match the following terms to the most appropriate definition by writing the correct letter in the space provided. Some terms may be used more than once. See text pp. 276-279.

A. type A+   D. type O−   G. hemolysis

B. type B+   E. Rh factor   H. kernicterus

C. type AB+   F. erythroblastosis fetalis

1. _____ the universal recipient
2. _____ the red blood cells of this blood type contain neither the A antigen nor the B antigen
3. _____ the plasma of this blood type contains both anti-A antibodies and anti-B antibodies
4. _____ the plasma of this blood type contains neither anti-A antibodies nor anti-B antibodies
5. _____ a person with this blood type can receive (by transfusion) type A, type B, type AB, and type O blood
6. _____ the universal donor
7. _____ a person with this blood type can receive (by transfusion) only type O− blood
8. _____ the administration of mismatched blood causes this serious condition
9. _____ the positive and negative signs (e.g., A+, A−) refer to this antigen
10. _____ severe hemolytic reaction in the fetus that is due to an antigen-antibody reaction involving the blood cells of the mother and fetus
11. _____ a serious neurologic complication of erythroblastosis fetalis that results in severe metal retardation
12. _____ blood type that contains only anti-B antibodies

13. _____ blood type that contains only anti-A antibodies

14. _____ a person with type A– blood can receive this type of blood

15. _____ a person with type B– blood can receive this type of blood

16. _____ blood type that includes the A antigen, B antigen, and the Rh factor

17. _____ consequence of administering type A+ blood to a patient who is type AB–

TELL A STORY

The Yellow Baby

Directions. Complete the story by using the words below. See text pp. 276-279.

erythroblastosis fetalis   Rh antigens   anti-RH antibodies

hemolysis   hyperbilirubinemia   A antigen

Ms. Billie Rubin (blood type A–) gave birth to Baby girl (type A+), a second daughter. Within 4 hours after birth, the baby appeared jaundiced; the jaundice intensified over the next 12 hours. What happened? Ms. Rubin has type A (–) blood and _____, having been sensitized from the first pregnancy. During the second pregnancy, the maternal antibodies slipped across the placenta into the baby and attacked the _____ of the baby's red blood cells, thereby causing agglutination and _____. The ruptured red blood cells release bilirubin causing _____ and jaundice. This condition is called _____.

MATCHING

Red Blood Cell Review with the Anemias

Directions. Match the following terms to the most appropriate definition by writing the correct letter in the space provided. Some terms may be used more than once. See text pp. 267-270, 276-278.

A. hemolytic anemia

B. folic acid deficiency anemia

C. pernicious anemia

D. sickle cell anemia

E. iron deficiency anemia

F. aplastic anemia

G. anemia of chronic renal (kidney) failure

1. _____ due to impaired function of the parietal cells in the stomach; they are unable to secrete intrinsic factor

2. _____ reticulocytes are usually absent

3. _____ a hereditary anemia that causes the red blood cells to form a rigid crescent shape

4. _____ endemic in a low-income population

5. _____ a diabetic with end-stage renal disease (diabetic nephropathy)

6. _____ anemia that characterizes erythroblastosis fetalis

7. _____ a megaloblastic anemia that is treated with vitamin B_{12} injections

8. _____ treated with ferrous sulfate

Student Name _____

9. _____ an infant who drinks only whole milk for his first year of life is likely to develop this type of anemia

10. _____ often accompanied by granulocytopenia and thrombocytopenia

11. _____ the most painful of the anemias

12. _____ myelosuppression

13. _____ anemia associated with occult blood [(+) guaiac test on stools]

14. _____ anemia that is characterized by jaundice

15. _____ the lack of intrinsic factor impairs the absorption of extrinsic factor

16. _____ a megaloblastic anemia that is commonly seen in pregnant women and patients with alcoholism

17. _____ the anemia most often associated with kernicterus

18. _____ a hypochromic microcytic anemia that is often caused by a chronic slow bleeding lesion

19. _____ often seen in a cancer patient who is being treated with powerful cytotoxic drugs and radiation

20. _____ following a severe hemorrhage, a person will experience this type of anemia

PART II: PUTTING IT ALL TOGETHER

MULTIPLE CHOICE

Directions. Choose the best answer.

1. Polymorphs (polys), segs, and band cells are
   a. platelets that become sticky and form a plug.
   b. erythrocytes that carry oxygen throughout the body.
   c. neutrophils.
   d. antibody-secreting agranulocytes.

2. Which of the following is a true statement?
   a. Most clotting factors are synthesized in the liver.
   b. Erythropoietin is secreted by the bone marrow.
   c. Prothrombin is synthesized by the kidney.
   d. The liver combines thrombin with vitamin K to make prothrombin.

3. Myelosuppression
   a. diminishes the numbers of blood cells.
   b. causes a deficiency of clotting factors.
   c. causes hypoprothrombinemia and a prolonged prothrombin time.
   d. activates plasminogen.

4. Vasospasm, platelet plug, and blood coagulation are most related to which process?
   a. agglutination
   b. phagocytosis
   c. cross-matching
   d. hemostasis

5. Carbon monoxide binds to
   a. granulocytes causing infection.
   b. hemoglobin causing hypoxia.
   c. platelets causing hypoxemia.
   d. bone marrow causing bleeding.

6. Which of the following descriptions is most related to an erythrocyte?
   a. a blood cell that participates in hemostasis
   b. a blood cell that becomes sticky upon activation
   c. a hemoglobin-containing cell that carries oxygen
   d. a phagocytic cell

7. Which of the following is the stimulus for the release of erythropoietin?

   a. elevated serum bilirubin
   b. lowered levels of oxygen
   c. increase in the amount of iron in the blood
   d. decrease in the synthesis of intrinsic factor

8. Which of the following is least descriptive of bilirubin?

   a. originates in hemoglobin
   b. liberated from heme
   c. stored in the liver and used in the synthesis of fibrinogen
   d. excreted in the bile

9. Erythroblastosis fetalis is most likely to occur in which of the following situations?

   a. mother is type A–; the baby is type A+
   b. mother is type B+; the baby is type B–
   c. mother is type B–; the baby is type B–
   d. mother is type AB+; the baby is type B+

10. Which combination is correct?

   a. hemolysis and cyanosis
   b. hypoxemia and jaundice
   c. hypoxemia and bleeding
   d. hypoprothrombinemia and bleeding

11. Granulocytopenia is most related to

   a. leukocytosis and fever.
   b. platelet deficiency and bleeding.
   c. neutropenia and infection.
   d. anemia and cyanosis.

12. Which of the following is not a function of plasma proteins?

   a. carry oxygen
   b. maintain blood volume
   c. transport hormones and substances such as bilirubin and drugs
   d. fight infection

13. Rapid hemolysis causes

   a. hypoxemia and flushing of the face.
   b. myelosuppression and bleeding.
   c. hyperbilirubinemia and jaundice.
   d. leukopenia and infection.

14. A person in chronic kidney failure is anemic because

   a. he cannot secrete adequate intrinsic factor.
   b. he cannot tolerate iron-rich foods.
   c. his kidneys do not secrete adequate erythropoietin.
   d. his diseased kidneys excrete folic acid.

15. Tissue plasminogen activator (tPA) is a drug that activates plasmin and therefore

   a. suppresses bone marrow activity.
   b. prevents the hepatic synthesis of prothrombin.
   c. blocks the hepatic use of vitamin K in the synthesis of prothrombin.
   d. dissolves clots.

16. Which of the following patients is most likely to benefit from an injection of vitamin K?

   a. patient with pernicious anemia
   b. patient who has iron deficiency anemia
   c. the granulocytopenic patient
   d. the hypoprothrombinemic patient

17. Albumin, globulins, and fibrinogen are all

   a. clotting factors.
   b. plasma proteins.
   c. anticoagulants.
   d. blood types.

18. Which condition is caused by venous stasis?

   a. bleeding
   b. thrombosis
   c. jaundice
   d. hemophilia

19. Which of the following is most likely to have a low reticulocyte count? The patient who

   a. is hypoprothrombinemic.
   b. has aplastic anemia.
   c. is hypoxic and cyanotic.
   d. is hyperbilirubinemic and jaundiced.

20. Who has a low hematocrit?

   a. Luke O'Cytosis
   b. Mac R. O'Phage
   c. Anne Emia
   d. Aunty C. O'agulant

Student Name _____

CASE STUDY

B.R., a 72-year-old widowed farmer, lives alone on a fixed income. He went to his physician complaining of being tired all the time. His diet consists primarily of tea and toast. A blood test revealed the following: a hemoglobin 9 g/dl, and a hematocrit of 27. He had a white blood cell (WBC) count of 9000/mm³ and a normal WBC differential count. His platelet count was 300,000/mm³. No other signs and symptoms were noted.

1. B.R.'s medical history and blood studies are most suggestive of which condition?

   a. hemophilia
   b. infection
   c. anemia
   d. platelet deficiency

2. What is the most likely cause of his medical condition?

   a. iron-poor diet
   b. drug-induced hemolysis
   c. thrombocytopenia
   d. infection

3. Which blood studies support the diagnosis?

   a. abnormal WBC count
   b. abnormal platelet count
   c. abnormally low hemoglobin and hematocrit
   d. elevated hematocrit

4. What is the cause of the fatigue (feeling tired all the time)?

   a. excessive phagocytic activity
   b. overstimulation of the bone marrow
   c. reduced oxygenation of the tissues
   d. bleeding

5. Which of the following blood studies ruled out an underlying infection?

   a. hematocrit
   b. hemoglobin
   c. normal WBC and WBC differential counts
   d. platelet count

PART III: CHALLENGE YOURSELF!

GROUPS AND PUZZLE

1. Which group is incorrect?

   a. Blood types: A, B, AB, O
   b. Clotting factors: prothrombin, fibrinogen, hemophilic factor
   c. Types of anemia: iron-deficiency, pernicious, sickle cell
   d. WBCs: granulocytes, agranulocytes, thrombocytes

2. Which group is incorrect?

    a. Results of myelosuppression: granulocytopenia, aplastic anemia, thrombocytopenia
    b. Types of anemia: iron-deficiency, pernicious, sickle cell
    c. Anticoagulants: heparin, Coumadin, plasmin, tPA
    d. Antigens: A, B, Rh factor

3. Which group is incorrect?

    a. Antigens: A, B, Rh factor
    b. Steps in hemostasis: blood vessel spasm, platelet plug, coagulation
    c. Plasma proteins: albumin, fibrinogen, platelets
    d. Results of myelosuppression: granulocytopenia, aplastic anemia, thrombocytopenia

PUZZLE

Hint: "Why the Yellow Fellow"?

Directions. Perform the following functions on the Sequence of Words below. When all the functions have been performed, you are left with word(s) that are related to the hint. Record your answer below.

Functions: remove the following

1. another name for the red blood cell

2. refers to bone marrow depression

3. the granulocytic white blood cell that is highly phagocytic

4. the anticoagulant that acts as an antithrombin agent

5. the organ that synthesizes erythropoietin

6. a vitamin K–dependent clotting factor

7. a deficiency of platelets that causes bleeding

8. the breakdown of red blood cells

9. the protein that fills the red blood cell and is concerned with the transport of oxygen

10. the ratio of the formed elements of the blood to the total blood volume

11. the organ that synthesizes prothrombin

Sequence of Words

LIVERHEMATOCRITPROTHROMBINHYPERBILIRUBINEMIATHROMBOCYTOPENIAMY
ELOSUPPRESSIONERYTHROCYTEHEMOLYSISCAUSESHEMOGLOBINNEUTROPHILKID
NEYJAUNDICEHEPARIN

Answer: _____

16

Anatomy of the Heart

Answer Key: Textbook page references are provided as a guide for answering these questions. A complete answer key was provided for your instructor.

Objectives

1. Describe the location of the heart.

2. Name the three layers and covering of the heart.

3. Explain the function of the heart as two separate pumps.

4. Identify the four chambers of the heart.

5. Explain the functions of the four heart valves.

6. Describe blood flow through the heart.

7. List the vessels that supply blood to the heart.

8. Identify the major components of the heart's conduction system.

PART I: MASTERING THE BASICS

MATCHING

Location, Layers, and Chambers of the Heart

Directions. Match the following terms to the most appropriate definition by writing the correct let-ter in the space provided. Some terms may be used more than once. See text pp. 283-287.

A. endocardium
B. pericardium
C. atria
D. ventricles
E. epicardium
F. angina pectoris
G. right atrium

H. coronary arteries
I. left atrium
J. right ventricle
K. myocardial infarction
L. coronary veins
M. myocardium
N. base

O. left ventricle
P. great vessels
Q. precordium
R. apex
S. pericardial cavity
T. cardiology

1. __B__ sling-like structure that supports the heart
2. __H__ delivers oxygenated blood to the myocardium CORONARY ARTERIES
3. __A__ smooth, shiny, innermost lining of the heart
4. __G__ chamber that receives unoxygenated blood from the venae cavae (R) ATRIUM
5. __J__ chamber that pumps unoxygenated blood to the lungs through the pulmonary artery (R) VENTRICLE
6. __P__ term that includes the venae cavae, pulmonary artery, pulmonary veins, and aorta
7. __D__ primary pumping chambers of the heart VENTRICLES
8. __I__ chamber that receives oxygenated blood from the lungs through four pulmonary veins (L) ATRIUM
9. __E__ outermost layer of the heart
10. __O__ chamber that pumps oxygenated blood into the systemic circulation (L) VENTRICLE
11. __O__ the myocardium is the thickest in this chamber (L) VENTRICLE
12. __K__ death of the heart muscle caused by occlusion of a coronary artery
13. __C__ receiving chambers of the heart ATRIA
14. __L__ drains unoxygenated blood from the myocardium
15. __F__ chest pain usually caused by impaired flow of blood through the coronary arteries
16. __Q__ area on the anterior chest that overlies the heart and great vessels
17. __H__ the LAD, also called the *widow-maker*
18. __O__ hardest-working chamber LEFT VENTRICLE
19. __M__ layer of the heart that contains the contractile proteins, actin and myosin
20. __B__ the epicardium is part of this structure
21. __N__ upper flat portion of the heart that is located at the level of the second rib
22. __S__ collection of fluid or blood in this space causes an external compression of the heart (called *cardiac tamponade*)

Student Name _____

23. ___S___ space between the epicardium and the parietal pericardium
24. ___T___ study of the heart
25. ___K___ heart attack
26. ___R___ lower pointed end of the heart that is located at the level of the fifth intercostal space

READ THE DIAGRAM

Blood Flow Through the Heart

Directions. Referring to the figure, write the correct number in the spaces below. See text p. 287.

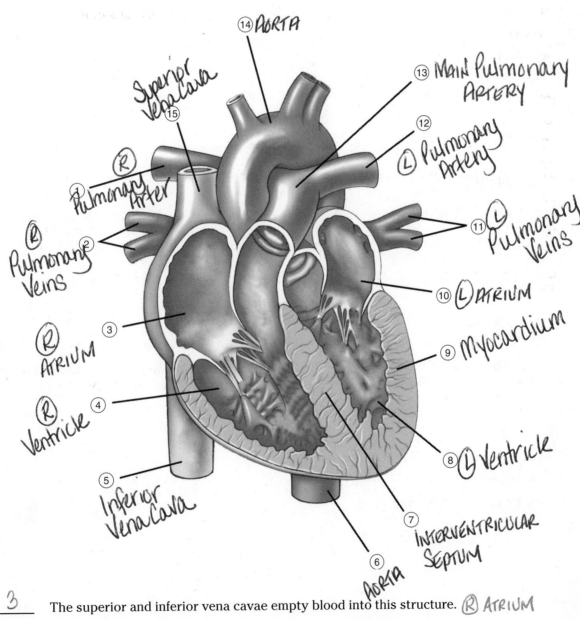

1. ___3___ The superior and inferior vena cavae empty blood into this structure. ® ATRIUM
2. ___14___ The left ventricle pumps blood into this structure. AORTA

3. __13__ The right ventricle pumps blood into this structure.

4. __10__ The pulmonary veins empty blood into this structure.

5. __7__ This separates the two pumping chambers.

6. __10__ , __8__ The bicuspid valve separates these two ~~structures~~ *chambers*. (L)A ; (L)V

7. __10__ , __8__ The mitral valve separates these two structures.

8. __8__ The aortic valve separates the aorta from this ~~structure~~ *chamber* (L) VENTRICLE

9. __13__ The pulmonic valve separates the right ventricle from this structure. PULMONARY ARTERY

10. __3__ , __4__ The tricuspid valve separates these two structures. (R)A ; (R)V.

11. __4__ Blood flows through the tricuspid valve into this chamber. (R)VENTRICLE

12. __13__ Blood is pumped through the pulmonic valve into this structure.

13. __8__ Blood flows through the mitral valve into this chamber. (L)VENTRICLE

14. __13__ Blood is pumped through the right semilunar valve into this structure.

15. __3__ Blood flows through the right AV valve from this chamber.

16. __8__ Blood flows through the left AV valve into this structure.

17. __10__ An incompetent mitral valve allows the retrograde flow of blood from the left ventricle into this structure.

18. __4__ A stenotic (narrowed) pulmonic valve causes hypertrophy of the muscle of this chamber.

19. __13__ An incompetent right semilunar valve allows the retrograde flow of blood from this structure into the right ventricle.

20. __8__ A stenotic left semilunar valve causes hypertrophy of the myocardium of this chamber.

COLORING

Directions. Color or mark the appropriate areas on the illustration on the previous page as indicated below.

1. Color all the structures that carry oxygenated blood **red**.

2. Color all the structures that carry unoxygenated blood **blue**.

3. Color the ventricular myocardium **yellow**.

4. Put an **X** over each AV valve.

5. Place a **Y** over each semilunar valve.

Student Name _____

MATCHING

Heart Valves and Sounds

Directions. Match the terms to the most appropriate definition by writing the correct letter in the space provided. Some terms may be used more than once. See text pp. 288-290.

A. tricuspid valve   E. pulmonic valve   I. chordae tendineae

B. bicuspid valve   F. aortic valve   J. S_1

C. murmurs   G. left ventricle   K. S_2

D. valvular stenosis   H. incompetent valve   L. gallop rhythm

✓ 1. __E__ semilunar valve through which blood leaves the right ventricle

2. __A__ atrioventricular valve on the right side of the heart

✓ 3. __B__ called the *mitral valve*   Bicuspid

4. __H__ leaky valve that allows backflow of blood

5. __J__ the first heart sound (lubb)

✓ 6. __F__ exit valve that sees only oxygenated blood

7. __I__ tough bands that attach the AV valves to the ventricular walls

8. __D__ refers to the narrowing of a valve

9. __L__ extra heart sounds (S_3, S_4) that sound like a racing horse

10. __F__ valve that prevents the backflow of blood into the left ventricle

11. __J__ heart sound created by the closure of the AV valves at the beginning of ventricular contraction

12. __B__ entrance valve that sees only oxygenated blood

13. __B__ valve that prevents the backflow of blood from the left ventricle

14. __B__ atrioventricular valve between the left atrium and the left ventricle

15. __E__ exit valve that sees only unoxygenated blood

16. __E__ valve that prevents the backflow of blood from the pulmonary artery

17. __K__ heart sound created by the closure of the semilunar valves at the beginning of ventricular relaxation

18. __F__ semilunar valve through which blood leaves the left ventricle

19. __C__ abnormal heart sounds caused by valvular disease

20. __A__ entrance valve that sees only unoxygenated blood

COMPLETE THE TABLE

Blood Flow

Directions. Complete the tables by filling in the names of the chambers and great vessels as blood flows through the heart. Example: Blood flows from the right atrium → right ventricle → pulmonary artery. See text pp. 290-291.

From →	To →	To
right atrium	right ventricle	pulmonary artery
pulmonary capillaries	pulmonary veins	left atrium
Left Atrium	Left Ventricle	aorta
Pulmonary veins	left atrium	Left Ventricle
venae cavae	Right Atrium	Right Ventricle
left atrium	Left Ventricle	AORTA
Pulmonary artery	pulmonary capillaries	Pulmonary veins
right Ventricle	main pulmonary artery	left pulmonary artery

Student Name _____

MATCHING

Conduction System

Directions. Match the terms to the most appropriate definition by writing the correct letter in the space provided. Some terms may be used more than once. See text pp. 293-296.

A. AV node
B. SA node
C. Purkinje fibers
D. QRS complex
E. tachycardia

F. normal sinus rhythm (NSR)
G. bundle of His
H. ectopic focus
I. ventricular fibrillation
J. electrocardiogram (ECG)

K. P wave
L. P-R interval
M. bradycardia
N. T wave

1. __I__ life-threatening dysrhythmia that causes the ventricular myocardium to quiver in an uncoordinated and ineffective way

2. __B__ pacemaker of the heart   *SA Node*

3. __M__ heart rate below 60 beats per minute   *bradycardia*

4. __G__ specialized conduction tissue in the interventricular septum; divides into the right and left branches   *– Bundle of His*

5. __B__ place where the electrical signal normally arises   *SA Node*

6. __A__ the electrical signal spreads from the conduction tissue in the atria to this structure   *AV Node*

7. __H__ area outside the SA node that gives rise to an electrical signal

8. __C__ these fast-conducting fibers spread the electrical signal throughout the ventricular wall   *Purkinje fibers*

9. __J__ record of the electrical activity of the heart (a heart chart)   *EKG*

10. __E__ heart rate greater than 100 beats per minute   *TACHYCARDIA*

11. __K__ ECG deflection that indicates atrial depolarization

12. __D__ ECG deflection that indicates ventricular depolarization

13. __N__ ECG deflection that represents ventricular repolarization

14. __L__ ECG recording that represents the time it takes for the electrical signal to travel from the SA node to the ventricles

15. __D__ electrical event that stimulates ventricular myocardial contraction

16. __K__ electrical event that stimulates atrial contraction

17. __L__ lengthening of this time indicates heart block

18. __F__ electrical activity appears normal and the signal arises within the SA node   *NORMAL SINUS RHYTHM*

√READ THE DIAGRAM

Conduction System

Directions. Referring to the figure, enter the numbers in the blanks. See text p. 294.

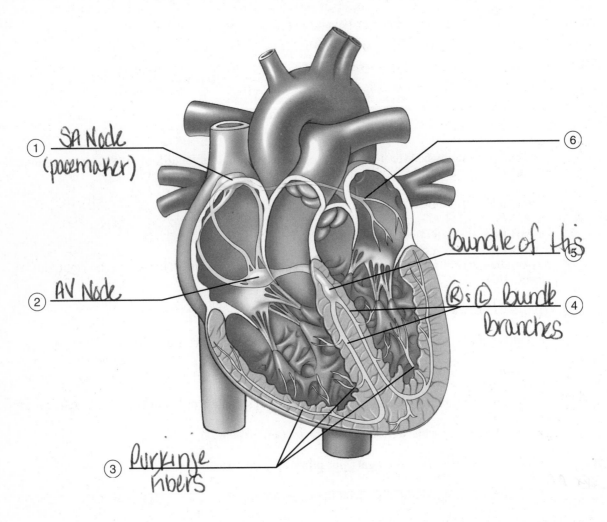

1. ___1___   pacemaker of the heart
2. ___5___   specialized conduction tissue in the interventricular septum; divides into the right and left branches
3. ___1___   where the electrical signal arises in normal sinus rhythm (NSR)
4. ___5,4___   a bundle
5. ___2___   the electrical signal spreads from the conduction tissue in the atria to this structure
6. ___3___   fast-conducting fibers that spread the electrical signal throughout the ventricular wall
7. ___2___   where the electrical signal arises in nodal rhythm
8. ___4___   electrical signal spreads to the Purkinje fibers   ℝ & 𝕃 bundle branches

from bundle of His

Student Name _____

ORDERING

√**Blood Flow Through the Heart**

Directions. Indicate by writing the correct term in the space provided. Two of the steps are given. See text p. 290.

bicuspid valve (mitral)   pulmonary capillaries   aorta

right ventricle   left ventricle   tricuspid valve

pulmonary artery (main)   pulmonary arteries (right and   left atrium
                                  left)
pulmonary veins (four)   pulmonic semilunar valve
                                  right atrium
                                                                  aortic semilunar valve

1.   right atrium

2.   TRICUSPID VALVE

3.   RIGHT VENTRICLE

4.   PULMONIC SEMILUNAR VALVE

5.   PULMONARY ARTERY (MAIN)

6.   PULMONARY ARTERIES (Right & left)

7.   pulmonary capillaries

8.   PULMONARY VEINS

9.   LEFT ATRIUM

10. BICUSPID VALVE (MITRAL)

11. LEFT VENTRICLE

12. AORTIC SEMILUNAR VALVE

13. AORTA

PART II: PUTTING IT ALL TOGETHER

MULTIPLE CHOICE

Directions. Choose the correct answer.

1. Which of the following is not related to the location of the heart?

    a. thoracic cavity
    b. mediastinum
    c. pleural cavity
    d. precordium

2. Oxygenated blood is found in which structure?

    a. right ventricle
    b. right atrium
    c. pulmonary artery
    d. pulmonary veins

3. What is the cause of the heart sounds "lubb-dupp"?

    a. vibrations caused by closure of valves
    b. firing of the SA node
    c. movement of blood through the valves
    d. flow of blood through the coronary vessels

4. Which of the following is an example of a tachydysrhythmia?

    a. NSR
    b. heart rate of 85 beats/min
    c. heart rate of 40 beats/min
    d. rapid and irregular heart rate

5. Which of the following statements is true?

    a. The left ventricular myocardium pumps blood to the pulmonic circulation.
    b. The left ventricular myocardium is thicker than the right ventricular myocardium because it works harder.
    c. The right ventricular myocardium pumps blood to the systemic circulation.
    d. The right ventricular myocardium pumps blood into the aorta.

6. Blood flow through the coronary arteries is greatest

    a. when the semilunar valves are open.
    b. during ventricular contraction.
    c. when the AV valves are closed.
    d. during ventricular relaxation.

7. Cardiac enzymes (LDH, CK, AST) and troponin elevate

    a. whenever a person experiences angina.
    b. when myocardial cells are damaged and leak their contents.
    c. during ventricular contraction when coronary blood flow diminishes.
    d. in the presence of valvular dysfunction.

8. The AV node

    a. slows the electrical signal as it moves from the atrium to the ventricles.
    b. is the pacemaker of the heart.
    c. is located in the upper right atrium.
    d. sends the electrical signal to the SA node.

9. The precordium is

    a. located within the mediastinum.
    b. located within the pericardial space.
    c. the anterior chest overlying the heart and great vessels.
    d. the space within the chambers of the heart.

10. The mitral valve is

    a. a semilunar valve; sees oxygenated blood.
    b. the right AV valve.
    c. a cuspid valve that sees unoxygenated blood.
    d. a cuspid valve.

11. Which of the following statements is least descriptive of the ventricular myocardium?

    a. contraction and relaxation
    b. pumping chambers
    c. QRS complex
    d. location of the SA node

Student Name _____

12. A child has a large ventricular septal defect (VSD) and pulmonic valve stenosis. Which of the following statements is true?

    a. Blood flow through the heart is normal.
    b. Blood shunts from the left ventricle to the right ventricle and the child is acyanotic.
    c. Blood shunts from the right ventricle to the left ventricle and the child is acyanotic.
    d. Blood shunts from the right ventricle to the left ventricle and the child is cyanotic.

13. Which of the following is not descriptive of the defect described in the previous question?

    a. congenital
    b. right-to-left shunt
    c. cyanotic heart defect
    d. left-to-right shunt

14. Which of the following describes the left anterior descending artery and the circumflex artery?

    a. parts of the vena cava
    b. parts of the pulmonic circulation
    c. branches of the left coronary artery
    d. branches of the descending aorta

15. The Purkinje fibers

    a. send electrical signals to the bundle of His.
    b. are the specialized cells of the SA node.
    c. are rapid conduction fibers that supply the ventricular myocardium.
    d. are responsible for the P wave (ECG).

16. The P-R interval (ECG)

    a. is shortened in heart block.
    b. represents atrial depolarization.
    c. represents the time it takes the signal to travel from the atrium to the ventricles.
    d. represents ventricular depolarization.

17. Ventricular contraction is least effective during

    a. bradycardia.
    b. NSR.
    c. ventricular fibrillation.
    d. exercise.

18. Which of the following is responsible for the opening and closing of heart valves?

    a. oxygen saturation of the blood in the heart chambers
    b. hematocrit
    c. pressure within the heart chambers
    d. tugging on the cusps

19. Who has the slowest heart rate?

    a. Angi O'Plasty
    c. Brady Cardia
    b. Perry Cardium
    d. Anne Gina

CASE STUDY

M.S. went to bed about 11 PM after a busy evening of entertaining friends and family. He was awakened at 2 AM with chest pain that radiated to his left shoulder, arm, and fingers. His son took him to the emergency room, where he was immediately given O_2 by mask and nitroglycerin, a vasodilator drug. His chest pain was relieved in about 30 minutes. An ECG revealed evidence of myocardial ischemia but no evidence of a myocardial infarction. He was admitted to the cardiac intensive care unit for further evaluation.

1. Which of the following is the most likely cause of the pain?

    a. an insufficient amount of oxygen available to the myocardium
    b. constriction of the heart by a swollen pericardium
    c. an inflamed valve
    d. strain of the shoulder and arm muscles

2. Which of the following terms refers to chest pain?

    a. heart attack
    b. myocardial infarction
    c. angina pectoris
    d. myocardial necrosis

3. Which of the following explains why nitroglycerin helps relieve anginal pain?

    a. It deadens the sensory nerves in the heart.
    b. It decreases the amount of "pumping" work by the heart.
    c. It causes the heart muscle to tetanize.
    d. It dissolves blood clots.

PART III: CHALLENGE YOURSELF!

GROUPS AND PUZZLE

1. Which group is incorrect?

    a. semilunar valves: pulmonic, aortic
    b. atrioventricular valves: tricuspid, bicuspid, mitral
    c. structures that carry oxygenated blood: pulmonary artery, left ventricle, aorta
    d. layers of the heart: epicardium, myocardium, endocardium

2. Which group is incorrect?

    a. structures that carry unoxygenated blood: right ventricle, pulmonary artery, venae cavae
    b. abnormal heart rates: tachycardia, bradycardia, normal sinus rhythm
    c. parts of the conduction system: SA node, AV node, bundle of His, Purkinje fibers
    d. layers of the heart: epicardium, myocardium, endocardium

3. Which group is incorrect?

    a. structures that carry unoxygenated blood: right ventricle, pulmonary artery, venae cavae
    b. layers of the heart: epicardium, myocardium, endocardium
    c. parts of the conduction system: SA node, AV node, bundle of His, coronary sinus
    d. chambers of the heart: atria, ventricles

Student Name _____

PUZZLE

Hint: Achey Breaky Heart

Directions. Perform the following functions on the Sequence of Words below. When all the functions have been performed, you are left with word(s) that are related to the hint. Record your answer below.

Functions: remove the following

1. two semilunar heart valves
2. all AV (cuspid) heart valves (3)
3. three layers of the heart
4. heart's sling
5. two pumping chambers
6. parts of the conduction system (3)
7. the left ventricle ejects blood into this large artery
8. the right ventricle ejects blood into this artery
9. blood vessels that nourish the myocardium
10. chamber that receives oxygenated blood from the pulmonary veins

Sequence of Words

LEFTATRIUMEPICARDIUMSANODEPULMONARYARTERYAVNODEENDOCARDIUMAORTICMITRALLEFTVENTRICLEMYOCARDIUMACUTEMYOCARDIALINFARCTIONCORONARYARTERIESPULMONICRIGHTVENTRICLEAORTAHIS-PURKINJESYSTEMANGINAPECTORISTRICUSPIDPERICARDIUMBICUSPID

Answer: _____ *and* _____

Acute Myocardial Infarcation
Angina Pectoris

17

Function of the Heart

Answer Key: Textbook page references are provided as a guide for answering these questions. A complete answer key was provided for your instructor.

Objectives

1. Define cardiac cycle with respect to systole and diastole.

2. Define cardiac output and explain how changes in heart rate and/or stroke volume change cardiac output.

3. Describe the autonomic innervation of the heart.

4. Describe the effect of the Starling's law of the heart on myocardial contraction.

5. Describe the inotropic effect on myocardial contraction.

6. Define preload and explain how it affects cardiac output.

7. Define afterload and identify the major factors that determine afterload.

8. Define the special clinical vocabulary used to describe cardiac function.

9. Define heart failure and differentiate between right-sided and left-sided heart failure.

PART I: MASTERING THE BASICS

MATCHING

Myocardial Function

Directions. Match the terms to the most appropriate definition by writing the correct letter in the space provided. See text pp. 299-303.

A. cardiac output	D. stroke volume	G. Starling's law of the heart
B. systole	E. cardiac cycle	H. cardiac reserve
C. diastole	F. positive inotropic effect	I. heart rate

1. __F__ increase in the strength of myocardial contraction that occurs without stretching the heart

2. __G__ increase in the strength of myocardial contraction that occurs when the heart is stretched

3. __B__ phase of the cardiac cycle that refers to contraction of the heart muscle

4. __E__ sequence of events that occurs in the heart in one beat

5. __I__ beats/minute

6. __C__ coronary blood flow is greatest during this phase of the cardiac cycle

7. __A__ determined by heart rate × stroke volume

8. __A__ amount of blood pumped by the heart in one minute

9. __D__ 70 ml/beat

10. __H__ the capacity to increase cardiac output above the resting cardiac output

11. __B__ what the ventricles are "doing" when the AV valves are closed and the semilunar valves are open

12. __D__ amount of blood pumped by the ventricle per beat

13. __E__ its duration is 0.8 seconds with a normal resting heart rate

14. __C__ the phase of the cardiac cycle that refers to relaxation of the ventricles

15. __G__ ability of the myocardium to match venous return and cardiac output on a beat-to-beat basis

16. __C__ phase of the cardiac cycle that shortens most in response to tachycardia

17. __C__ what the ventricles are "doing" when the AV valves are open and the semilunar valves are closed

18. __A__ 5000 ml/min

Student Name _____

MATCHING

Autonomic Innervation of the Heart

Directions. Indicate if the following effects are due to sympathetic activity (S) or parasympathetic activity (P). See text pp. 300-305.

1. __S__ increases heart rate and stroke volume
2. __S__ is associated with the "fight-or-flight" response
3. __S__ increases cardiac output
4. __P__ also called *vagal activity*
5. __S__ causes a (+) chronotropic and (+) inotropic effect
6. __P__ excess activity causes bradycardia and heart block
7. __P__ causes a (–) chronotropic and (–) dromotropic effect
8. __S__ causes a racing and pounding heart
9. __P__ causes bradydysrhythmias
10. __S__ causes tachydysrhythmias
11. __S__ produces effects similar to epinephrine (Adrenalin) and dopamine
12. __P__ effects similar to a vagomimetic drug
13. __P__ the resting heart rate is dominated by this branch of the autonomic nervous system
14. __S__ increases force of myocardial contraction
15. __P__ digoxin slows the heart rate by stimulating this branch of the ANS

MATCHING

Electrical or Muscle Contraction

Directions. Indicate if the following are most related to the electrical signal or cardiac muscle contraction. Fill in the blank with either electrical (E) or contraction (C). See text pp. 299-303.

1. __C__ actin and myosin
2. __C__ inotropic effect
3. __E__ depolarization
4. __E__ QRS complex
5. __C__ stroke volume
6. __E__ T wave
7. __E__ repolarization
8. __C__ systole
9. __C__ sliding filaments
10. __C__ Starling's law of the heart
11. __E__ pacemaker
12. __C__ diastole
13. __E__ dysrhythmia
14. __E__ bundle of His
15. __C__ sarcomere
16. __E__ ectopic focus
17. __E__ ECG
18. __E__ Purkinje fibers

MATCHING

Heart Talk

Directions. Match the terms to the most appropriate definition by writing the correct letter in the space provided. Some words may be used more than once. See text pp. 303-305.

A. afterload	C. chronotropic effect	E. ejection fraction
B. inotropic effect	D. end diastolic volume	F. dromotropic effect

1. __D__   forms the basis of Starling's law of the heart
2. __E__   the percentage of the EDV that is pumped
3. __A__   the resistance or opposition to the flow of blood
4. __D__   the amount of blood in the ventricles at the end of its resting phase
5. __F__   change in the rate or speed that the cardiac impulse travels through the conduction system of the heart
6. __A__   an example is the aortic blood pressure
7. __D__   EDV
8. __D__   also called *preload*
9. __B__   change in myocardial contractile force that is not due to stretch
10. __C__   change in heart rate

MATCHING

Autonomic Receptors of the Heart

Directions. Indicate if the following effects are characteristics of the sympathetic nervous system (S) or the parasympathetic nervous system (P). See text pp. 305-306.

1. __S__   norepinephrine is the postganglionic neurotransmitter
2. __P__   activation of muscarinic receptors
3. __S__   activation of the beta$_1$ receptors
4. __P__   vagomimetic effects
5. __P__   acetylcholine is the postganglionic neurotransmitter
6. __P__   activation of cholinergic receptors

Student Name _____

MATCHING

Heart Failure

Directions. Indicate if the description is more characteristic of left-sided heart failure (L) or right-sided heart failure (R). See text pp. 306-308.

1. __L__   three-pillow dyspnea
2. __R__   hepatomegaly (enlarged liver), distended jugular veins (JVD), pedal edema
3. __L__   pulmonary edema
4. __R__   consequence of chronic lung disease such as emphysema and asthma
5. __L__   backup within the pulmonary capillaries causing water to accumulate in the lungs
6. __L__   cyanosis, dyspnea, orthopnea
7. __L__   most likely to say "I can't breathe."
8. __L__   most likely to develop in response to chronic systemic hypertension
9. __R__   cor pulmonale

PART II: PUTTING IT ALL TOGETHER

MULTIPLE CHOICE

Directions. Choose the correct answer.

1. Actin and myosin, striated and involuntary are descriptive terms for the

    a. valves.
    b. myocardium.
    c. pericardium.
    d. great vessels.

2. Seventy (70) ml/beat × 72 beats/minute is the amount of blood that determines

    a. ejection fraction.
    b. stroke volume.
    c. cardiac output.
    d. cardiac reserve.

3. Which of the following terms describes myocardial contraction and relaxation?

    a. depolarization and repolarization
    b. P wave and T wave
    c. systole and diastole
    d. tachycardia and bradycardia

4. Which of the following occurs during ventricular systole?

    a. Blood is pumped out of the ventricles.
    b. The ventricles fill with blood.
    c. The AV valves open.
    d. The semilunar valves close.

5. The heart drug digitalis stimulates the parasympathetic nerve that supplies the heart. What cardiac effect is expected?

    a. The valves open faster.
    b. The heart rate increases.
    c. The pulse increases.
    d. The heart rate slows.

6. Which of the following increases stroke volume?

    a. (+) chronotropic effect
    b. (+) dromotropic effect
    c. decreased EDV
    d. (+) inotropic effect

7. Stretching the heart causes the force of myocardial contraction to increase. This stretch effect is called

    a. (+) inotropic effect.
    b. cor pulmonale.
    c. Starling's Law of the Heart.
    d. cardiac tamponade.

8. A chronic elevation in afterload, as in systemic hypertension, is most likely to cause

    a. a left-to-right shunt.
    b. cor pulmonale.
    c. left ventricular hypertrophy.
    d. jugular vein distention (JVD).

9. If heart rate increases to 170 beats/minute

    a. the length of diastole decreases.
    b. coronary blood flow increases.
    c. EDV increases.
    d. preload increases.

10. An increase venous return of blood to the heart

    a. decreases EDV.
    b. increases preload.
    c. decreases cardiac output.
    d. decreases stroke volume.

11. Preload is most related to

    a. heart rate.
    b. Starling's Law of the Heart.
    c. an inotropic effect.
    d. SA node activity.

12. A drug, such as atropine, that blocks the muscarinic receptors is most likely to

    a. induce a severe bradycardia.
    b. cause a (−) dromotropic effect leading to heart block.
    c. increase heart rate.
    d. decreases cardiac output.

13. A β_1 adrenergic agonist

    a. causes bradycardia.
    b. increases cardiac output.
    c. decreases stroke volume.
    d. decreases ejection fraction.

14. Norepinephrine

    a. activates muscarinic receptors.
    b. is antagonized by muscarinic blockade.
    c. is a β_1 adrenergic agonist.
    d. blocks β_1 adrenergic receptors.

15. Blockade of the effects of acetylcholine (ACh) on the heart

    a. decreases cardiac output.
    b. increases heart rate.
    c. causes a prolongation of the P-R interval (heart block).
    d. causes bradydysrhythmias.

16. What happens when the actin and myosin in the ventricles form crossbridges?

    a. The valves open.
    b. The myocardium contracts.
    c. The heart enters the period of diastole.
    d. The ventricles fill with blood.

17. In order for the ventricles to fill, the

    a. AV valves must be closed.
    b. semilunar valves must be open.
    c. ventricles must be in diastole.
    d. chordae tendineae must be fully relaxed.

18. If the QRS complex does not develop, the

    a. heart develops a sustained muscle contraction (tetanizes).
    b. ventricular myocardium does not contract.
    c. ventricles contract at a rate that mimics that of the SA node.
    d. ventricular myocardium remains in systole and can't relax.

19. Which of the following is most likely to increase ejection fraction?

    a. vagal discharge
    b. activation of the muscarinic receptors
    c. blockade of the β_1 adrenergic receptors
    d. stimulation of the sympathetic nervous system

20. Which of the following is an age-related cardiac change?

    a. Resting heart rate increases to 90 beats per minute.
    b. Starling's Law of the Heart is lost.
    c. The sarcoplasmic reticulum loses its ability to store calcium.
    d. The heart muscle cannot respond as vigorously to the demands of exercise.

Student Name _____

CASE STUDY

> Mr. I. is 61-year-old male who was admitted to the ER because of a sudden and severe increase blood pressure (205/100 mm Hg). He was complaining of chest pain, a headache in the back of his head, and a sense of not feeling well. Mr. I. has a history of coronary artery disease and evidence of left ventricular hypertrophy on ECG. He admitted to poor drug compliance (omitting his blood pressure medication) for the past two weeks. He was subsequently treated with a calcium channel blocker drug that quickly reduced his blood pressure to 155/95 mm Hg. He was discharged and advised to lose weight, exercise, and resume his antihypertensive drug schedule.

1. Both the chest pain and the left ventricular hypertrophy are due to

   a. fluid accumulation in the pulmonary capillaries and alveoli.
   b. the increased afterload.
   c. pulmonary artery hypertension.
   d. accumulation of fluid in the pericardial space.

2. Which of the following drug effects decreases afterload?

   a. increased venous return
   b. reduction of blood pressure
   c. (+) inotropic effect
   d. (+) dromotropic effect

3. A calcium channel blocker slows heart rate and decreases force of myocardial contraction. Which of the following best describes these effects?

   a. vasopressor and diuresis
   b. (−) chronotropic effect and (−) inotropic effect
   c. (+) inotropic effect, decreased ejection fraction
   d. (−) dromotropic effect and diuresis

PART III: CHALLENGE YOURSELF

GROUPS AND PUZZLE

1. Which group is incorrect?

   a. receptors: alpha, beta, and muscarinic
   b. determinants of cardiac output: stroke volume, heart rate
   c. effects of sympathetic stimulation: (+) inotropic effect, (+) chronotropic effect
   d. words that affect the SA node: chronotropic effect, pacemaker, inotropic effect

2. Which group is incorrect?

   a. receptors: alpha, beta, and muscarinic
   b. determinants of cardiac output: stroke volume, heart rate
   c. effects of parasympathetic stimulation: (−) chronotropic effect, (−) inotropic effect
   d. words that affect the SA node: chronotropic effect, pacemaker, bradycardia

3. Which group is incorrect?

   a. receptors: alpha, beta, and diastole
   b. determinants of cardiac output: stroke volume, heart rate
   c. effects of parasympathetic stimulation: (−) chronotropic effect, bradycardia
   d. words that affect the SA node: chronotropic effect, pacemaker, tachycardia

PUZZLE

Hint: Ejection Fraction of 30%

Directions. Perform the following functions on the Sequence of Words below. When all the functions have been performed, you are left with word(s) that are related to the hint. Record your answer below.

Functions: remove the following

1. contractile proteins (2) found in the myocardium
2. phases of the cardiac cycle that refer to myocardial contraction and relaxation
3. electrical terms (2) that form the basis of the P wave, QRS complex, and T wave
4. parasympathetic nerve that supplies the SA and AV nodes
5. transmitters (2) of the autonomic nerves of the heart
6. determinants (2) of cardiac output
7. mechanisms (2) to change force of myocardial contraction
8. term that refers to a heart rate >100 beats/minute; term that refers to a heart rate of <60 beats/minute
9. terms (2) that refers to the amount of blood in the ventricles at the end of its resting phase
10. cholinergic and adrenergic receptors on the SA and AV nodes

Sequence of Words

INOTROPICEFFECT~~ENDDIASTOLICVOLUME~~BETA~~BRADYCARDIA~~NOREPINEPHRINE~~S~~ ~~TROKEVOLUMEMYOSIN~~HEARTFAILURE~~VAGUSDEPOLARIZATIONACTINDIASTOLESYS~~ ~~TOLEREPOLARIZATION~~ACETYLCHOLINE~~HEARTRATE~~STARLINGSLAWOFTHEHEART~~TA~~ ~~CHYCARDIA~~MUSCARINIC~~PRELOAD~~

Answer: _____

18

Anatomy of the Blood Vessels

Answer Key: Textbook page references are provided as a guide for answering these questions. A complete answer key was provided for your instructor.

Objectives

1. Describe the pulmonary and systemic circulations.

2. Describe the structure and function of arteries, capillaries, and veins.

3. List the three layers of tissue found in arteries and veins.

4. Explain the functions of conductance, resistance, exchange, and capacitance vessels.

5. List those major arteries of the systemic circulation that are branches of the ascending aorta, aortic arch, and descending aorta.

6. List the major veins of the systemic circulation.

7. Describe the following special circulations: blood supply to the head and brain, hepatic circulation, and fetal circulation.

PART I: MASTERING THE BASICS

MATCHING

Arrangement of Blood Vessels

Directions. Match the following terms to the most appropriate definition by writing the correct letter in the space provided. Some terms may be used more than once. See text pp. 313-316.

A. systemic circulation   D. venules   F. capillaries

B. veins   E. arteries   G. arterioles

C. pulmonary circulation

1. __E__ large blood vessels that carry blood away from the heart

2. __B__ capacitance vessels

3. __C__ the path of the blood from the right ventricle of the heart to the lungs and back to the left atrium

4. __F__ these tiny blood vessels are composed of a single layer of epithelium and therefore function as exchange vessels

5. __B__ blood vessels that carry blood back to the heart

6. __A__ the path of the blood from the left ventricle of the heart to the body cells and back to the right atrium

7. __G__ small arteries composed primarily of smooth muscle

8. __F__ vessels that connect the arterioles with the venules

9. __D__ small veins that drain the capillaries and converge to form large veins

10. __F__ exchange vessels

11. __G__ resistance vessels

12. __F__ the most numerous of the blood vessels

13. __B__ large vessels that contain valves

Student Name _____

MATCHING

Arteries

Directions. Match the following terms to the most appropriate definition by writing the correct let-ter in the space provided. Some terms may be used more than once. See text pp. 316-319.

A. celiac trunk
B. circle of Willis
C. coronary arteries
D. renal artery

E. internal carotid arteries
F. common iliac arteries
G. mesenteric arteries
H. dorsalis pedis artery

I. aorta
J. basilar artery
K. hepatic artery
L. left subclavian artery

1. __J__ the vertebral arteries pass upward from the subclavian arteries toward the back of the neck; they extend upward into the cranium and join to form this artery

2. __K__ a branch of the celiac trunk that supplies the liver

3. __I__ largest artery in the body; it arises from the left ventricle of the heart

4. __D__ artery that supplies the kidney

5. __G__ these arteries are branches of the abdominal aorta; they supply blood to most of the small intestine and part of the large intestine

6. __B__ an arrangement of arterial blood vessels found at the base of the brain

7. __H__ an extension of the anterior tibial artery that supplies the foot

8. __F__ the distal end of the abdominal aorta splits, or bifurcates, into this

9. __A__ short artery that divides into the gastric artery, splenic artery, and hepatic artery

10. __I__ large artery that is classified as ascending, arch, and descending

11. __I__ large artery that is classified as thoracic and abdominal

12. __C__ branches of the ascending aorta that supply the myocardium of the heart

13. __E__ arteries that ascend on the anterolateral aspect of the neck; supply the circle of Willis

14. __L__ branch of the aortic arch that supplies the left shoulder and upper arm

15. __E__ name that means *heavy sleep* or *stupor*

MATCHING

Veins

*Directions. Match the following terms to the most appropriate definition by writing the correct let-
ter in the space provided. Some words may be used more than once. See text pp. 319-321.*

A. superior vena cava	E. renal vein	H. great saphenous vein
B. inferior vena cava	F. subclavian vein	I. median cubital vein
C. jugular veins	G. portal vein	J. femoral vein
D. hepatic veins		

1. __H__ located in the lower extremity; it is the longest vein in the body
2. __J__ large deep vein in the thigh that enters the pelvis as the external iliac vein
3. __b__ the common iliac vein continues as this vein
4. __A__ this large vein drains the head, shoulders, and upper extremities and empties the blood into the right atrium
5. __G__ formed from the union of the superior mesenteric vein and the splenic vein
6. __C__ drain the head
7. __b__ large vein that returns blood to the right atrium from all the regions below the diaphragm
8. __E__ drains blood from the kidney and empties it into the inferior vena cava
9. __G__ large vein that carries blood from the digestive organs to the liver
10. __D__ drains the liver and empties blood into the vena cava
11. __F__ receives blood from the axillary vein and the external jugular vein
12. __H__ long superficial vein often "borrowed" for cardiac bypass surgery
13. __I__ vein that joins the cephalic and basilic veins
14. __I__ arm vein that is commonly used to withdraw a sample of blood

MATCHING

Fetal Circulation

*Directions. Match the following terms to the most appropriate definition by writing the correct let-
ter in the space provided. Some terms may be used more than once. See text pp. 324-326.*

A. foramen ovale	C. ductus arteriosus	E. placenta
B. ductus venosus	D. umbilical cord	

1. __D__ structure that carries three blood vessels (two arteries and one vein); it connects the mother with the fetus
2. __A__ hole in the interatrial septum that allows fetal blood to shunt from the right atrium to the left atrium
3. __E__ place for maternal-fetal exchange of nutrients, gases, and waste

Student Name _____

4. __B__   structure that connects the umbilical vein with the fetal inferior vena cava; it shunts blood past the fetal liver

5. __C__   short tube that connects the fetal pulmonary artery with the aorta

6. __E__   structure that serves as lungs for the fetus

7. __C__   failure of this opening to close after birth creates a left-to-right shunt between the aorta and the pulmonary artery

8. __A__   failure of this opening to close after birth creates a left-to-right shunt between the atria

TRACE A DROP OF BLOOD

Directions. Refer to Figures 18-4, 18-5, 18-6, 18-7, and 18-8 in the textbook and using the words below, fill in the blanks. The words can be used more than once. (L is left, R is right.) See text pp. 316-321.

circumflex artery	R atrium	superior vena cava
L atrium	R popliteal vein	L femoral artery
R axillary vein	L femoral vein	R brachial artery
abdominal aorta	inferior vena cava	pulmonary artery
R subclavian artery	R common iliac vein	R brachiocephalic vein

1. Pulmonary artery → pulmonary capillaries → pulmonary veins → _(L) Atrium_ → left ventricle → ascending aorta → aortic arch → right brachiocephalic artery → _(R)Subclavian artery_ → right axillary artery → _(R)brachial artery_ → right radial artery

2. Thoracic aorta → _abdominal aorta_ → left common iliac artery → left external iliac artery → _(L) femoral artery_ → left popliteal artery → left anterior tibial artery → left dorsalis pedis artery

3. Right internal jugular vein → _(R)brachiocephalic vein_ → superior vena cava → right atrium → right ventricle → _pulmonary artery_ → pulmonary capillaries → left atrium

4. Right radial vein → right brachial vein → _(R)Axillary vein_ → right subclavian vein → right brachiocephalic vein → _Superior Vena Cava_ → right atrium

5. Right anterior and posterior tibial veins → _(R)popliteal vein_ → right femoral vein → right external iliac → _(R)common iliac vein_ → inferior vena cava → right atrium

6. Left saphenous vein → _(L)femoral vein_ → left external iliac vein → left common iliac vein → _Inferior vena cava_ → right atrium

7. Ascending aorta → left coronary artery → _circumflex artery_ → walls of the left heart → cardiac veins → cardiac sinus → _(R) Atrium_

TRACE A DROP OF BLOOD, AGAIN

Directions. Using the words below, fill in the blanks. The words can be used more than once. See text pp. 316-326.

umbilical vein	R ventricle	umbilical arteries
inferior vena cava	R common carotid artery	hepatic vein
foramen ovale	ductus arteriosus	R atrium
circle of Willis	pulmonary veins	pulmonary artery
L common carotid artery	portal vein	superior mesenteric vein

1. _umbilical vein_ → ductus venosus → inferior vena cava → right atrium → _foramen ovale_ → left atrium → left ventricle → ascending aorta → descending aorta → _umbilical arteries_ → placenta

2. _____ → ductus venosus → _____ → right atrium → right ventricle → pulmonary artery → _____ → thoracic aorta → abdominal aorta → internal iliac arteries → _____ → placenta

3. Pulmonary capillaries → _____ → left atrium → left ventricle → ascending aorta → aortic arch → _____ → left internal carotid artery → basilar artery → _____

4. Ascending aorta → aortic arch → right brachiocephalic artery → _____ right internal carotid artery → _____

5. Splenic vein → _____ hepatic sinusoids → hepatic vein → _____ → right atrium → _____ → pulmonary artery

6. _____ → portal vein → hepatic sinusoids → _____ → inferior vena cava → _____ → right ventricle → _____ → pulmonary capillaries → pulmonary veins → left atrium → left ventricle → aorta

PART II: PUTTING IT ALL TOGETHER

MULTIPLE CHOICE

Directions. Choose the correct answer.

1. Blood that is a bright red color (as opposed to a bluish-red color)
   a. is always found in arteries.
   b. is never found in veins.
   c. is oxygenated.
   d. has a high concentration of carbaminohemoglobin.

2. About 70% of the blood volume is located in which structures?
   a. veins
   b. capillaries
   c. resistance vessels
   d. arteries

3. Arterioles have a lot of smooth muscle that allows them to
   a. act as exchange vessels.
   b. store large amounts of blood.
   c. contract and relax, thereby affecting blood vessel diameter.
   d. prevent a backward flow of blood.

4. The internal carotid and vertebral arteries
   a. are called the *circle of Willis*.
   b. empty blood into the subclavian arteries.
   c. supply oxygenated blood the arteries of the brain.
   d. drain cerebrospinal fluid from the brain.

Student Name _____

5. The purpose of the ductus arteriosus is to

   a. oxygenate blood.
   b. bypass the fetal lungs.
   c. bypass the fetal liver.
   d. conduct blood to the fetal pulmonary capillaries.

6. The foramen ovale

   a. is found in the interventricular septum.
   b. bypasses the fetal liver.
   c. shunts blood from the pulmonary artery to the aorta.
   d. shunts blood from the right heart to the left heart.

7. Failure of the ductus arteriosus to close after birth

   a. causes immediate death.
   b. decreases blood flow to the lungs.
   c. causes blood to shunt from the pulmonary artery to the aorta.
   d. causes a left-to-right shunt.

8. Which of the following is a correct statement about the fetal circulation?

   a. There is one umbilical artery.
   b. There are two umbilical veins.
   c. The umbilical veins carry unoxygenated blood.
   d. There is one umbilical vein that carries oxygenated blood.

9. The jugulars

   a. carry unoxygenated blood from the brain.
   b. are part of the hepatic portal circulation.
   c. are exchange blood vessels.
   d. are resistance vessels.

10. Most often atherosclerosis of a carotid artery causes

   a. facial flushing.
   b. cyanosis and breathlessness.
   c. cognitive impairment.
   d. cold, pale extremities.

11. Right-sided heart failure is most likely to cause

   a. pulmonary edema.
   b. cyanosis and orthopnea.
   c. jugular vein distention (JVD).
   d. cough, air hunger, and restlessness.

12. The portal vein

   a. supplies most of the oxygenated blood to the liver.
   b. carries blood from the digestive organs directly to the inferior vena cava.
   c. carries blood that is rich is digestive end-products to the liver.
   d. receives blood from the hepatic veins.

13. The superior mesenteric and splenic veins

   a. receive unoxygenated blood from the portal vein.
   b. bypass the liver and empty blood into the inferior vena cava.
   c. merge to form the portal vein.
   d. deliver blood to the stomach and intestines to aid in digestion.

14. Ascites, portal hypertension, and esophageal varices are conditions caused by

   a. elevated portal vein pressure.
   b. hyperbilirubinemia and jaundice.
   c. chronic hypoxia.
   d. elevated plasma ammonia.

15. The subclavian veins

   a. are found only in the fetal circulation.
   b. are part of the hepatic portal circulation.
   c. are part of the circle of Willis.
   d. empty blood into the brachiocephalic veins.

16. What is true of both the anterior tibial artery and the dorsalis pedis arteries?

   a. both run parallel to the great saphenous
   b. both are part of the hepatic portal circulation
   c. both are found in the lower extremities
   d. both contain valves

17. The basilar artery

   a. delivers blood to the circle of Willis.
   b. is part of the celiac axis.
   c. supplies oxygenated blood to the liver.
   d. is a branch of the aortic arch that becomes the vertebral artery as it ascends the posterior neck region.

CASE STUDY

Polly Phagia is a type 2 diabetic with neuropathy and atherosclerosis of the blood vessels of the lower extremities. She is admitted to your unit because of an area of her great toe that appears blackened.

1. What is the concern (if any) of the blackened toe?

    a.   There is no concern; we can assume she stubbed her toe.
    b.   The poor circulation starves the tissue of oxygen and nutrients, causing gangrene.
    c.   She must be in excruciating pain.
    d.   She has lost her sense of balance.

2. What is the effect of poor arterial circulation to the feet (as is true with many diabetics)?

    a.   The feet feel warm.
    b.   The dorsalis pedis pulse may be undetectable.
    c.   The feet sweat excessively.
    d.   The feet appear red.

PART III: CHALLENGE YOURSELF!

GROUPS AND PUZZLE

1. Which of the following is incorrect?

    a.   types of blood vessels: conductance, resistance, exchange, capacitance
    b.   layers of the blood vessel walls: intima, media, adventitia
    c.   divisions of the aorta: ascending, arch, descending
    d.   names of veins: jugular, portal, circle of Willis

2. Which of the following is incorrect?

    a.   types of blood vessels: arteries, capillaries, veins
    b.   names of arteries: aorta, circle of Willis, jugular, basilar
    c.   types of blood vessels: conductance, resistance, exchange, capacitance
    d.   layers of the blood vessel walls: intima, media, adventitia

3. Which of the following is incorrect?

    a.   types of blood vessels: arteries, capillaries, veins
    b.   names of veins: jugular, portal, vena cava
    c.   types of blood vessels: conductance, resistance, exchange, capacitance
    d.   layers of the blood vessel walls: intima, media, myocardium

Student Name _____

PUZZLE

Hint: Vain Jane Complains of Vein Pain

Directions. Perform the following functions on the Sequence of Words below. When all of the functions have been performed, you are left with word(s) that are related to the hint. Record your answer below.

Functions: remove the following

1. main vein that drains the brain
2. main vein named superior and inferior
3. longest vein in the leg
4. large deep vein in the thigh
5. large vein that delivers blood to the liver
6. vein that merges with the superior mesenteric vein to form the portal vein
7. vein that drains the jugular vein
8. chamber of the heart that receives blood from the venae cavae
9. veins that carry oxygenated blood from the lungs to the left heart
10. a vein in the arm

Sequence of Words

VENAECAVAEJUGULARSPLENICPORTALSUBCLAVIANTHROMBOPHLEBITISFEMORALS
APHENOUSPULMONARYBASILICRIGHTATRIUM

Answer: _____

19

Functions of the Blood Vessels

Answer Key: Textbook page references are provided as a guide for answering these questions. A complete answer key was provided for your instructor.

Objectives

1. Explain how the blood vessels act as a delivery system.

2. Describe the factors that determine blood pressure.

3. Explain the baroreceptor reflex.

4. Describe the factors that determine capillary exchange.

5. Describe mechanisms of edema formation.

6. Explain how the blood vessels respond to changing body needs.

7. Describe the role of the blood vessels in the regulation of body temperature.

PART I: MASTERING THE BASICS

MATCHING

Directions. Use the following words to fill in the blanks. Some words are used more than once. See text pp. 330-340.

A. capillaries   D. edema   F. arterioles

B. blood pressure   E. capillary filtration pressure   G. ischemia

C. albumin

1. __F__ resistance vessels
2. __A__ exchange vessels
3. __F__ determines systemic vascular resistance (SVR)
4. __G__ it's cool: pulselessness, pallor, pain. paresthesia, paralysis
5. __B__ determined by cardiac output × SVR
6. __C__ determines plasma oncotic pressure
7. __G__ impaired blood flow to a tissue or organ
8. __C__ a deficiency of this plasma protein causes edema
9. __B__ determined by stroke volume × heart rate × systemic vascular resistance
10. __D__ abnormal collection of fluid
11. __B__ the force exerted by the blood against the walls of the blood vessels
12. __E__ the outward pushing pressure within the exchange vessels

MATCHING

Blood Pressure

Directions. Match the following terms to the most appropriate definition by writing the correct letter in the space provided. Some terms may be used more than once. See text pp. 330-337.

A. hypotension   F. systemic vascular resistance (SVR)   K. postural hypotension

B. normal blood pressure   L. diastolic pressure

C. sphygmomanometer   G. brachial   M. Korotkoff sounds

D. pulse pressure   H. pulse   N. mean arterial blood pressure (MABP)

E. hypertension   I. systolic pressure

     J. vasopressors

1. __K__ a sudden drop in blood pressure when the person moves from a lying to a standing position; often causes dizziness and fainting
2. __H__ vibrations of the blood vessel walls that reflect heart rate
3. __M__ the noise heard through the stethoscope when blood pressure is measured
4. __F__ in addition to cardiac output, this determines blood pressure

Student Name _____

5. __I__ the pressure in the arteries at the peak of ventricular contraction

6. __G__ the artery most commonly used to measure blood pressure

7. __D__ the difference between the systolic reading and the diastolic reading

8. __A__ this is most likely to be caused by a massive peripheral vasodilation

9. __N__ diastolic blood pressure + 1/3 pulse pressure

10. __B__ blood pressure of 120/80 mm Hg

11. __J__ hormones or drugs that increase blood pressure

12. __E__ this is most likely to be caused by intense peripheral vasoconstriction

13. __C__ a device used to measure blood pressure

14. __E__ blood pressure reading of 160/95 mm Hg

15. __A__ blood pressure reading of 75/40 mm Hg; a "shocky" blood pressure

16. __L__ the pressure in the arteries during ventricular relaxation

17. __M__ silence...tap...tap...tap... muffle

18. __I__ the top number of a blood pressure reading

19. __L__ the bottom number of a blood pressure reading

READ THE DIAGRAM

Baroreceptor Reflex

Directions. Refer to Figure 19-6 in the textbook and use the words to fill in the blanks. See text pp. 336-337.

A. red	D. sympathetic	G. vagus
B. green	E. medulla oblongata	H. parasympathetic
C. carotid sinus	F. spinal cord	I. aortic arch

1. __C__ and __I__ location of the blood pressure receptors

2. __B__ the color of the nerves that carry sensory information to the CNS

3. __A__ color of the nerves that carry parasympathetic responses to the SA and AV nodes

4. __A__ color of the nerves that carry vagal responses to the heart

5. __A__ color of the nerve that tells the heart rate to increase in response to a sudden decline in blood pressure

6. __E__ origin of the parasympathetic fibers that transmit responses to the heart

7. __D__ name of the nerve that transmits responses to the arterioles

8. __F__ origin of the sympathetic fibers that transmit responses to the heart and arterioles

9. __G__ another name for the parasympathetic nerve that supplies the heart

ʟ

MATCHING

Blood Pressure Readings

Directions. Refer to the following blood pressure readings and fill in the blanks below. See text pp. 330-337.

A. 115/75 mm Hg

B. 210/105 mm Hg

C. 72/48 mm Hg

1. __C__ blood pressure that causes a reflex tachycardia

2. __C__ blood pressure that may require a vasopressor drug

3. __A__ normotension

4. __B__ blood pressure that may require an antihypertensive drug such as a calcium channel blocker

5. __B__ blood pressure that may require the use of an α_1 adrenergic antagonist

6. __C__ blood pressure caused by hemorrhage

7. __B__ blood pressure that may result from excess catecholamines such as epinephrine

8. __B__ blood pressure that may be caused by intense sympathetic discharge

9. __B__ this person has a pulse pressure of 105 mm Hg

10. __C__ this person has a mean arterial blood pressure (MABP) of 56 mm Hg

11. __A__ this person has a pulse pressure of 40

12. __A__ this person has a mean arterial blood pressure of 89 mm Hg

13. __B__ blood pressure that is most likely to cause a stroke or brain attack

14. __C__ blood pressure that is most likely to underperfuse the heart muscle causing chest pain and the possibility of a myocardial infarction (MI)

15. __B__ this blood pressure is most likely to be treated with a drug that causes peripheral vasodilation

MATCHING

Nervous Stimulation of the Heart and Blood Vessels

Directions. Indicate whether the following are due to the firing of sympathetic nerves (S) or parasympathetic nerves (P) by writing the correct letter in the space provided. See text pp. 300-303, 333-337.

1. __P__ decrease in heart rate

2. __P__ same as a vagal discharge

3. __S__ (+) inotropic effect

4. __S__ increased blood pressure

5. __S__ increased force of myocardial contraction

6. __S__ increased cardiac output

7. __S__ increased systemic vascular resistance

8. __S__ (+) chronotropic effect

Student Name _____

9. __P__ (−) dromotropic effect
10. __P__ most likely to cause heart block
11. __S__ most likely to cause tachycardia
12. __P__ most likely to cause bradycardia
13. __S__ mimics the effects of the catecholamines

PART II: PUTTING IT ALL TOGETHER

MULTIPLE CHOICE

Directions. Choose the correct answer.

1. Reflex tachycardia is most likely to develop in response to

   a. pedal edema.
   b. blunting of the baroreceptor reflex by a β_1 adrenergic blocker.
   c. sudden decline in blood pressure.
   d. expanded blood volume.

2. A person with poor skin turgor is most likely have this condition.

   a. edema
   b. jaundice
   c. cyanosis
   d. dehydration

3. An increase in systemic vascular resistance is most likely to cause which condition?

   a. increased heart rate
   b. increased blood pressure
   c. hypotension
   d. anemia

4. A vasopressor substance

   a. thins the blood.
   b. decreases heart rate.
   c. decreases cardiac output.
   d. increases blood pressure.

5. What is the stimulus for the baroreceptor reflex ?

   a. change in blood pH
   b. pulse rate
   c. oxygen saturation of blood in the aortic arch and carotid sinus
   d. stretch of receptors located in several of the large arteries

6. What is the effect of stimulation of the sympathetic nerve?

   a. peripheral vasodilation
   b. decreases cardiac output
   c. decreases heart rate
   d. increases blood pressure

7. Which of the following is regulated by the renin-angiotensin-aldosterone system?

   a. blood pressure
   b. plasma protein synthesis
   c. plasma levels of calcium
   d. blood glucose

8. During strenuous exercise, the percentage of blood flow to which structure is greatly increased?

   a. kidney
   b. digestive tract
   c. skeletal muscles
   d. reproductive system

9. Which condition occurs if the amount of water filtered out of the capillary exceeds the amount of water reabsorbed into the capillary?

   a. dehydration
   b. poor skin turgor
   c. edema
   d. inflammation

10. Which of the following contributes to an increased venous return of blood during exercise?

    a. increased capillary filtration pressure
    b. increased oncotic pressure
    c. effect of the skeletal muscle pump
    d. activation of erythropoiesis by the bone marrow

11. What measurement do you need to calculate pulse pressure?

    a. hematocrit... 45%
    b. heart rate... 72 beats/minute
    c. pulse deficit... 5 beats
    d. blood pressure... 120/80 mm Hg

12. What measurement do you need to calculate mean arterial pressure?

    a. pulse pressure... 40 mm Hg
    b. heart rate... 72 beats/minute
    c. pulse deficit... 5 beats
    d. blood pressure... 120/80 mm Hg

13. Which of the following is least true of vaso-constriction?

    a. caused by sympathetic discharge
    b. decreases cardiac output and blood pressure
    c. increases afterload
    d. moves blood from the venous circulation to the arterial circulation

14. A person has a history of essential hypertension; he has been taking flu medication for the past 3 weeks. The flu medicine contains phenylephrine, an α_1 adrenergic agonist. What adverse effect might the person experience?

    a. stuffy nose from congested nasal mucous membrane
    b. further elevation in blood pressure
    c. drowsiness and fatigue
    d. constipation and bloating

15. Which of the following cannot be determined from a blood pressure reading of 130/72 mm Hg?

    a. systolic reading
    b. diastolic reading
    c. pulse
    d. pulse pressure

16. Which of the following makes the capillaries ideal exchange vessels?

    a. large area for diffusion
    b. slow velocity of blood flow
    c. thin capillary membrane
    d. all of the above

17. A collar that exerts pressure over the baroreceptors may

    a. cause hypotension and fainting.
    b. cause a hypertensive crisis and stroke.
    c. cause cerebral ischemia and loss of consciousness.
    d. inhibit venous drainage causing jugular vein distension.

18. What is most likely to "tent"?

    a. the valves of the large veins of the legs
    b. the capillaries that contain an expanded blood volume
    c. the skin of a dehydrated person
    d. the heart of an exercising person

19. Plasma oncotic pressure

    a. pulls water into the capillary from the interstitium.
    b. pushes water out of the capillary into the interstitium.
    c. pushes water from the interstitium into the cells.
    d. pumps K^+ into the cells.

20. What is the effect of an age-related stiffening of the blood vessel walls?

    a. anemia
    b. increased blood pressure
    c. increased cardiac output
    d. decreased diastolic pressure

21. Who is "Mr. Resistance"?

    a. Cappy Lary
    b. Angie O'Plasty
    c. Art Eriole
    d. Basil R.

CASE STUDY

C.L. went to the physician for his annual physical. Although he had no symptoms, his blood pressure was elevated at 160/95 mm Hg. He was advised to lose weight, begin an exercise program, and take medication for his blood pressure.

1. What is the goal of therapy?

    a. decrease the systolic reading to 90 mm Hg
    b. decrease the pulse pressure to 10
    c. decrease both the systolic and diastolic pressures
    d. achieve a heart rate of 60 beats/minute

2. Which type of pill would act as an antihypertensive agent? One that

    a. stimulates the sympathetic nerves.
    b. increases peripheral resistance.
    c. causes a vasopressor effect.
    d. causes vasodilation, thereby decreasing systemic vascular resistance.

PART III: CHALLENGE YOURSELF!

GROUPS AND PUZZLE

1. Which of the following is incorrect?

    a. hypertensive blood pressure readings: 172/95 mm Hg, 165/90 mm Hg, 147/88 mm Hg
    b. hypotensive blood pressure readings: 110/64 mm Hg, 80/65 mm Hg, 72/58 mm Hg
    c. determinants of blood pressure: heart rate, stroke volume, vascular resistance
    d. types of blood vessels: conductance, resistance, exchange, capacitance

2. Which of the following is incorrect?

    a. hypertensive blood pressure readings: 172/95 mm Hg, 165/90 mm Hg, 147/88 mm Hg
    b. hypotensive blood pressure readings: 82/48 mm Hg, 65/52 mm Hg, 72/58 mm Hg
    c. determinants of blood pressure: heart rate, stroke volume, pulse pressure
    d. types of blood vessels: conductance, resistance, exchange, capacitance

PUZZLE

Hint: Why Is Al Bumin a Swell Fellow?

Directions. Perform the following functions on the Sequence of Words below. When all the functions have been performed, you are left with word(s) that are related to the hint. Record your answer below.

Functions: remove the following

1. five Ps of ischemia

2. top and bottom blood pressure numbers

3. name of the resistance vessels and exchange vessels

4. difference between the systolic and diastolic blood pressure

5. three determinants of blood pressure

6. effects of straining at stools

7. location (2) of baroreceptors

Sequence of Words

CAPILLARIESCAROTIDSINUSPAINONCOTIC(SWELLING)SYSTOLICPRESSUREDIA
STOLICPRESSUREHEARTRATEVALSALVAMANEUVERONCOTICARTERIOLESSTROKEV
OLUMEPRESSUREAORTICARCHPULSELESSNESSPALLORPARESTHESIASPULSEPRES
SURESYSTEMICVASCULARRESISTANCEPARALYSIS

Answer: _____

20

Lymphatic System

Answer Key: Textbook page references are provided as a guide for answering these questions. A complete answer key was provided for your instructor.

Objectives

1. List three functions of the lymphatic system.

2. Describe the composition and flow of lymph.

3. Describe the four lymphoid organs: lymph nodes, tonsils, thymus gland, and spleen.

4. State the location of the following lymph nodes: cervical nodes, axillary nodes, and inguinal nodes.

PART I: MASTERING THE BASICS

MATCHING

Organs of the Lymphatic System

Directions. Match the following terms to the most appropriate definition by writing the correct letter in the space provided. Some terms may be used more than once. See text pp. 346-351.

A. subclavian veins

B. thoracic duct

C. right lymphatic duct

D. lymph

E. lymph nodes

F. thymosin

G. thymus

H. spleen

1. _____ a gland located in the upper thorax; it is most active during early life and is concerned with the processing and maturation of T lymphocytes

2. _____ tissue fluid that enters the lymphatic vessels

3. _____ lymph from the right arm and the right side of the head and thorax drain into this large duct

4. _____ hormone secreted by the thymus gland

5. _____ acts as a storage reservoir for blood

6. _____ small, pea-shaped structures that filter lymph as it flows through lymphatic vessels

7. _____ abdominal organ that resembles a large lymph node; it filters blood rather than lymph

8. _____ most of the lymph of the body drains into this large duct

9. _____ contains red pulp and white pulp; it is the largest lymphoid organ in the body

10. _____ the right lymphatic duct and the thoracic duct empty lymph into these blood vessels

MATCHING

Lymph Nodes and Tonsils

Directions. Match the following terms to the most appropriate definition by writing the correct letter in the space provided. See text pp. 348-350.

A. lingual

B. cervical

C. inguinal

D. pharyngeal

E. axillary

F. palatine

1. _____ lymph nodes that drain the upper extremities, shoulders, and breast areas

2. _____ small masses of lymphoid tissue (tonsils) located at the opening of the oral cavity into the pharynx

3. _____ tonsils located at the back of the tongue

4. _____ lymph nodes that drain the head and neck area

5. _____ tonsils located near the opening of the nasal cavity in the upper pharynx; also called the *adenoids*

6. _____ lymph nodes that drain lymph from the lower extremities and the groin area

Student Name _____

DRAW IT

Directions. Using this illustration, draw in the following structure.

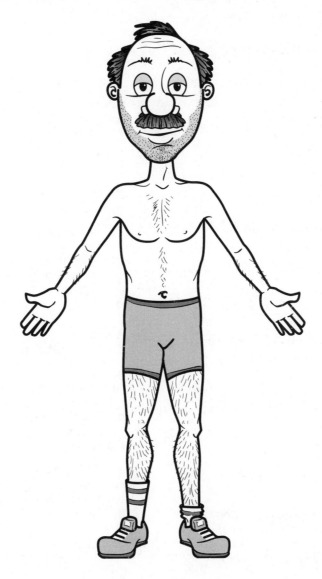

1. The thymosin-secreting gland that involutes during puberty.

2. The organ that functions as a giant lymph node; called the *graveyard of the red blood cells.*

3. Draw a chain of inguinal lymph nodes.

4. Draw a chain of cervical lymph nodes.

5. Draw a chain of axillary lymph nodes.

6. Place an X over the lymph nodes that may be affected with tonsillitis.

7. Place a Y over the lymph nodes that are often biopsied/removed during a mastectomy.

8. Place a Z over the lymph nodes that may be removed/radiated in a patient with a pelvic tumor.

9. Shade in the area (light blue) that is drained by the thoracic duct.

10. Shade in the area (yellow) that is drained by the right lymphatic duct.

PART II: PUTTING IT ALL TOGETHER

MULTIPLE CHOICE

Directions. Choose the correct answer.

1. The lymph nodes, thymus gland, spleen, and tonsils

    a. are confined to the thoracic cavity.
    b. are confined to the ventral cavity.
    c. are lymphoid organs.
    d. synthesize erythrocytes.

2. Which of the following best describes a tonsil?

    a. a partially encapsulated lymph node
    b. inguinal lymph nodes
    c. salivary gland
    d. goblet cell

3. The adenoids

    a. are tonsils.
    b. are located within the inguinal region.
    c. are located within the mediastinum.
    d. involute (shrivel) with age.

4. What is the name of the substance from which lymph is made?

    a. aqueous humor
    b. cerebrospinal fluid
    c. hemoglobin
    d. tissue fluid

5. If the spleen becomes overactive, it prematurely removes platelets from the circulation, causing thrombocytopenia. As a result, what condition is the person likely to develop?

    a. excessive bleeding
    b. jaundice
    c. infectious mononucleosis
    d. lymphedema

6. A tonsillectomy is most often performed on which set of tonsils?

    a. adenoids
    b. palatine
    c. pharyngeal
    d. lingual

7. Which of the following is least related to the spleen?

    a. destroys and phagocytoses old, worn-out red blood cells
    b. lymphoid organ
    c. a vital organ (can't live without the spleen)
    d. LUQ

8. A radical mastectomy with lymph node dissection is likely to cause

    a. lymphedema.
    b. thrombocytopenia and bleeding.
    c. granulocytopenia and infection.
    d. platelet deficiency.

9. Cancer of the breast first metastasizes to the

    a. adenoids.
    b. spleen.
    c. axillary lymph nodes.
    d. thymus gland.

10. The thoracic duct

    a. empties lymph into the subclavian veins.
    b. receives lymph from the entire right side of the body.
    c. contains blood.
    d. is the main duct within the spleen.

Student Name _____

CASE STUDY

M.K. is an 18-year-old college freshman. During exam week he developed a high fever; sore throat; general malaise; a productive cough; and a small, painful lump in his neck. A physician diagnosed him as having the flu and prescribed bedrest, aspirin, and fluids.

1. What is the most likely cause of the painful lump?

   a. A neck muscle was sprained during a bout of coughing.
   b. A lymph node became inflamed as it was fighting the infection.
   c. The painful lump is unrelated to the infection and is probably due to cancer of the lymph nodes.
   d. The painful lump is a blood-filled cyst.

2. Which of the following is most descriptive of the painful lump?

   a. adenoid
   b. malignant neoplasm
   c. cervical lymph node
   d. thoracic duct

3. What should eventually happen to the painful lump?

   a. It should metastasize.
   b. It should continue to grow and eventually require surgical removal.
   c. As the infection clears up, the lump and pain should disappear.
   d. The surface of the lump should ulcerate, thereby allowing for drainage of pus.

PART III: CHALLENGE YOURSELF!

GROUPS AND PUZZLE

1. Which group is incorrect?

   a. collection of lymph nodes: cervical, axillary, inguinal
   b. tonsils: palatine, pharyngeal, lingual
   c. lymphoid organs: lymph nodes, tonsils, thymus gland, spleen
   d. large lymphatic ducts: right lymphatic duct, thoracic duct, adenoids

2. Which group is incorrect?

   a. collection of lymph nodes: cervical, axillary, inguinal
   b. tonsils: palatine, pharyngeal, thymosin
   c. lymphoid organs: lymph nodes, tonsils, thymus gland, spleen
   d. large lymphatic ducts: right lymphatic duct, thoracic duct

PUZZLE

Hint: Aching Adenoids

Directions. Perform the following functions on the Sequence of Words below. When all of the functions have been performed, you are left with word(s) that are related to the hint. Record your answer below.

Functions: remove the following

1.   the three sets of tonsils

2.   the large lymph node that resides in the LUQ

3.   the two large lymphatic ducts that drain into the subclavian veins

4.   three groups of lymph nodes

5.   lymphoid organ located within the mediastinum; involutes with age

Sequence of Words

THYMUSGLANDCERVICALPALATINESPLEENINGUINALRIGHTLYMPHATICDUCTLINGUA
LTONSILLITISPHARYNGEALAXILLARYTHORACICDUCT

Answer: _____

21

Immune System

Answer Key: Textbook page references are provided as a guide for answering these questions. A complete answer key was provided for your instructor.

Objectives

1. Differentiate between specific and nonspecific immunity.

2. Describe the process of phagocytosis.

3. Explain the causes of the signs of inflammation.

4. Explain the role of fever in fighting infection.

5. Explain the role of T cells in cell-mediated immunity.

6. Explain the role of B cells in antibody-mediated immunity.

7. Differentiate between genetic immunity and acquired immunity.

8. Describe naturally and artificially acquired active and passive immunity.

9. Identify the steps in the development of anaphylaxis.

PART I: MASTERING THE BASICS

MATCHING

Nonspecific Immunity

Directions. Match the following terms to the most appropriate definition by writing the correct letter in the space provided. Some terms may be used more than once. See text pp. 356-359.

A. inflammation	D. phagocytes	G. fever
B. natural killer (NK) cells	E. protective proteins	H. reflexes
C. mechanical barriers	F. chemical barriers	

1. _____ classic symptoms are redness, heat, swelling, and pain

2. _____ caused by pyrogens

3. _____ special type of lymphocyte that acts nonspecifically to kill certain cells

4. _____ regulated by a hypothalamic thermostat

5. _____ describes the white blood cells, particularly the neutrophils and monocytes, wandering around the body and engaging in cellular eating

6. _____ treated with an antipyretic drug such as aspirin

7. _____ examples are sneezing, coughing, and vomiting

8. _____ examples are lysozyme found in tears and hydrochloric acid in the stomach

9. _____ examples are interferons and complement proteins

10. _____ examples are intact skin and mucous membranes

11. _____ examples are tears, saliva, and perspiration

Student Name _____

MATCHING

Specific Immunity

Directions. Match the following terms to the most appropriate definition by writing the correct letter in the space provided. Some terms may be used more than once. See text pp. 359-363.

A. antigen

B. antigen presentation

C. immunotolerance

D. lymphocytes

E. lymphokines

F. plasma cell

G. cell-mediated immunity

H. autoimmune disease

I. macrophage

J. clone

K. thymus gland

L. antibody-mediated immunity

M. bone marrow

N. agglutination

1. _____ T and B cells

2. _____ a foreign substance, usually a large protein, that provokes a specific response

3. _____ the cell-to-cell contact by which T cells attack antigens directly

4. _____ also called *humoral immunity*

5. _____ recognition of self

6. _____ the cell responsible for antigen presentation

7. _____ attack against self

8. _____ type of immunity associated with immunoglobulins

9. _____ site where T cells mature and differentiate

10. _____ site where B cells mature and differentiate

11. _____ a group of identical cells formed from the same parent cell

12. _____ reacts with an antibody to cause clumping

13. _____ an allergen

14. _____ substances secreted by activated T cells that enhance phagocytic activity

15. _____ a subgroup of the B cell clone that produces antibodies

16. _____ ability of the macrophage to push an antigen to its surface

READ THE DIAGRAM

Immunoglobulin E Hypersensitivity Reaction

Directions. Referring to the illustration, fill in the blanks with the numbers. See text p. 365.

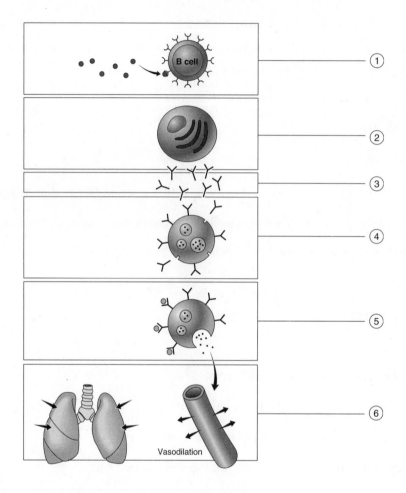

1. _____ illustrates the consequences of histamine release
2. _____ antigens bind to the receptors on the B cell
3. _____ antigens bind to IgE antibodies on the mast cells
4. _____ histamine is released from mast cell
5. _____ antibodies are secreted
6. _____ the intact mast cell with its IgE antibodies
7. _____ B cell clone that secretes antibodies
8. _____ illustrates an anaphylaxis-induced dyspnea (difficulty in breathing)
9. _____ a circulating lymphocyte
10. _____ illustrates an anaphylaxis-induced hypotension
11. _____ illustrates the reason that the mast cell bursts

MATCHING

Types of Immunity

Directions. Match the following terms to the most appropriate definition by writing the correct letter in the space provided. Some terms may be used more than once. See text pp. 362-365.

A. titer

B. immunization

C. genetic immunity

D. secondary response

E. primary response

F. naturally acquired active immunity

G. naturally acquired passive immunity

H. artificially acquired active immunity

I. artificially acquired passive immunity

1. _____ inborn, inherited, innate, or species immunity

2. _____ a type of immunity achieved by getting an injection of gamma globulin

3. _____ an infant receives antibodies (IgA) from her mother while breastfeeding

4. _____ level of antibodies in the blood

5. _____ immunization achieved by the injection of attenuated measles virus

6. _____ an infant received antibodies (IgG) from his mother while in utero

7. _____ immunization achieved by injection of a toxoid

8. _____ the type of immunity stimulated by a vaccine

9. _____ the type of natural immunity that mandates you will not get the disease if exposed to the virus as an adult because you had the disease as a child

10. _____ initial response of the plasma cells to an antigen

11. _____ related to a booster shot

12. _____ the type of immunity that mandates you will not get Dutch elm disease from your tree

13. _____ also called *vaccination*

14. _____ antitoxins, antivenoms

PART II: PUTTING IT ALL TOGETHER

MULTIPLE CHOICE

Directions. Choose the correct answer.

1. When a pathogen causes redness, heat, swelling, and pain it is called

   a. chemotaxis.
   b. diapedesis.
   c. an anaphylactic reaction.
   d. infection.

2. Which of the following is most related to pus?

   a. hyperbilirubinemia and jaundice
   b. phagocytosis and infection
   c. autoimmune disease
   d. thrombocytopenia and bleeding

3. Leukocytes "go" to the site of infection. Which of the following is descriptive of this activity?

   a. fever and flushing
   b. histamine and urticaria
   c. diapedesis and chemotaxis
   d. mitosis and neoplasia

4. Which of the following is most descriptive of a Kupffer cell? It

   a. is a helper T cell.
   b. is a "fixed" macrophage located within the liver.
   c. is a memory cell.
   d. secretes antibodies.

5. Which of the following speeds up the recognition of an antigen (allergen) when it is introduced for a second and third time?

   a. suppressor T cell
   b. neutrophil
   c. phagocyte
   d. memory cell

6. What is the term that refers to the capacity of our bodies to protect against pathogens and other foreign agents?

   a. diapedesis
   b. chemotaxis
   c. complement fixation
   d. immunity

7. Which of the following includes mechanical barriers, chemical barriers, and certain reflexes?

   a. specific defense mechanisms
   b. third line of defense
   c. nonspecific defense mechanisms
   d. second line of defense

8. The "big- eating" fixed phagocytes located in the liver, spleen, and lymph nodes

   a. are called natural killer cells.
   b. are B cells.
   c. are macrophages.
   d. develop in response to a specific antigen.

9. Which of the following is an immune system stimulator?

   a. use of anticancer drugs
   b. use of steroids
   c. aging
   d. administration of a "booster shot"

10. Fever-producing substances (pyrogens)

    a. are released by phagocytes as they perform their tasks.
    b. cause the release of histamine.
    c. are called *interferons*.
    d. immunoglobulins.

11. Interferons are

    a. proteins secreted by a cell infected by a virus that prevent further viral replication.
    b. complement proteins.
    c. called *IgE antibodies*.
    d. secreted by T cells.

12. Your own cells and secretions are recognized by your body as nonantigenic. What is this recognition-of-self called?

    a. immunity
    b. immunocompetence
    c. immunotolerance
    d. autoimmunity

13. Antibody-mediated immunity

    a. is achieved by B cells.
    b. operates by cell-to-cell combat.
    c. always results in anaphylaxis.
    d. is achieved by natural killer cells.

CASE STUDY

While romping through the fields one day, Aunty Bea was attacked and stung by an angry swarm of bees. Knowing that she was allergic to bee venom, her friends rushed her to the nearest emergency room. By the time she reached the emergency room, Bea's lips and tongue were swollen and she was unable to speak. Her breathing was labored and she was becoming cyanotic. She was immediately given an injection of epinephrine and steroids, intubated, and placed on oxygen.

1. What process is involved in the allergic response?

    a. the release of lysozyme
    b. the release of histamine in response to IgE antibodies
    c. only the nonspecific defense mechanisms
    d. only the cell-mediated immune response

2. Why was Bea dyspneic (having difficulty breathing)?

    a. The bee venom caused widespread vasodilation.
    b. The bee venom paralyzed olfactory receptors in the nasal passages.
    c. The swelling of the respiratory passages blocked the movement of air in and out of the lungs.
    d. She was too anxious to breathe normally.

3. Why was the oxygen administered? To

    a. block the release of additional histamine.
    b. activate the steroid.
    c. neutralize the bee venom.
    d. correct the hypoxemia and cyanosis.

4. Why was epinephrine administered? To

    a. dilate the respiratory passages.
    b. neutralize the bee venom.
    c. lower the blood pressure.
    d. help the liver degrade the histamine.

5. Which of the following is true of histamine?

    a. is released from plasma cells.
    b. causes constriction of the respiratory passages and decreases the flow of air.
    c. causes vasoconstriction and an increase in blood pressure.
    d. should be administered intravenously to combat the allergic response to the bee venom.

PART III: CHALLENGE YOURSELF

GROUPS AND PUZZLE

1. Which group is incorrect?

    a. first line of defense: skin, tears, sneezing
    b. mechanical barriers: skin, mucous membrane
    c. protective proteins: interferons, NK cells, T cells
    d. signs of inflammation: redness, heat, swelling, pain

2. Which group is incorrect?

    a. chemical barriers: tears, saliva, stomach acid
    b. protective proteins: interferons, complement proteins
    c. nonspecific immunity: inflammation, NK cells, fever, protective proteins, T cells
    d. T cell subgroups: killer T cells, helper T cells, suppressor T cells, memory cells

3. Which group is incorrect?

    a. specific immunity: B cells, T cells, NK cells
    b. mechanical barriers: skin, mucous membrane
    c. chemical barriers: tears, saliva, stomach acid
    d. immunoglobulins: IgA, IgM, IgG, IgE

PUZZLE

Hint: Inflammation: Rubor, Calor, Tumor, Dolor

Directions. Perform the following functions on the Sequence of Words below. When all of the functions have been performed, you are left with word(s) that are related to the hint. Record your answer below.

Functions: remove the following

1. immunoglobulins (4)

2. cells (2) that comprise the specific immune response

3. protective proteins (2)

4. convey active immunity (2)

5. conveys passive immunity (1)

6. antibody-secreting B cells

7. four members of the T cell clone

8. the immediate-onset and most severe allergic reaction

9. fever-producing

10. pus-producing

11. inflammation caused by a pathogen

12. means hives

Sequence of Words

PYOGENICREDNESSINFECTIONHEATPYROGENICKILLERSWELLINGGAMMAGLOBULI
NINTERFERONSTCELLCOMPLEMENTPROTEINURTICARIASUPPRESSORIgATOXOIDIgM
MEMORYVACCINEIgAPAINIgEBCELLPLASMACELLSHELPERANAPHYLAXIS

Answer: _____, _____, _____, _____

22

Respiratory System

Answer Key: Textbook page references are provided as a guide for answering these questions. A complete answer key was provided for your instructor.

Objectives

1. Describe the structure and functions of the organs of the respiratory system.

2. Trace the movement of air from the nostrils to the alveoli.

3. Describe the role of pulmonary surfactants.

4. Describe the relationship of Boyle's law to ventilation.

5. Explain how respiratory muscles affect thoracic volume.

6. List three conditions that make the alveoli well-suited for the exchange of oxygen and carbon dioxide.

7. List lung volumes and capacities.

8. Describe common variations and abnormalities of breathing.

9. Explain the neural and chemical control of respiration.

PART I: MASTERING THE BASICS

MATCHING

Structures of the Respiratory System

Directions. Match the following terms to the most appropriate definition by writing the correct let-ter in the space provided. Some terms may be used more than once. See text pp. 370-377.

A. larynx   E. paranasal sinuses   I. bronchi

B. trachea   F. lungs   J. glottis

C. nasal cavities   G. alveoli   K. esophagus

D. pharynx   H. bronchioles   L. carina

1. __B__ called the *windpipe,* it is a strong cartilaginous tube that conducts air to and from the lungs

2. __D__ respiratory structure that communicates with the middle ear by the eustachian tube

3. __A__ the Adam's apple or thyroid cartilage is most associated with this structure

4. __K__ the epiglottis directs food and water from the respiratory passages into this structure

5. __D__ called the *throat*

6. __A__ called the *voice box* because it contains the vocal cords

7. __L__ the point at which the trachea bifurcates (splits); the area is extremely sensitive and elicits coughing when stimulated (as in suctioning with a catheter)

8. __B__ located between the larynx and the bronchi and in front of the esophagus

9. __D__ composed of three parts: naso-, oro-, and laryngo-

10. __B__ large tube that splits into bronchi

11. __H__ these small structures located within the bronchial tree are composed primarily of smooth muscle

12. __G__ the exchange of the respiratory gases between the air and blood occurs here

13. __F__ large, soft, cone-shaped organs that contain the respiratory passages and pulmonary capil-laries; they fill most of the thoracic cavity

14. __H__ because of smooth muscle, this structure can contract and relax, thereby causing constric-tion and dilation

15. __C__ the olfactory receptors are located within these cavities

16. __E__ mucus drains into the nasal cavities from these structures located in the head

17. __I__ the trachea splits into the right and left

18. __H__ small respiratory passages that deliver oxygen to the alveoli

19. __G__ structures partially encircled by the pulmonary capillaries

20. __H__ called the *resistance vessels*

21. __G__ structures that contain surfactants

22. __C__ separated by the nasal septum

23. __J__ the space between the vocal cords

24. __G__ respiratory structure with the largest cross-sectional area; designed for gas exchange

Student Name _____

READ THE DIAGRAM

Structures of the Respiratory Tract

Directions. Referring to the illustration, fill in the blanks with the numbers. See text pp. 370-377.

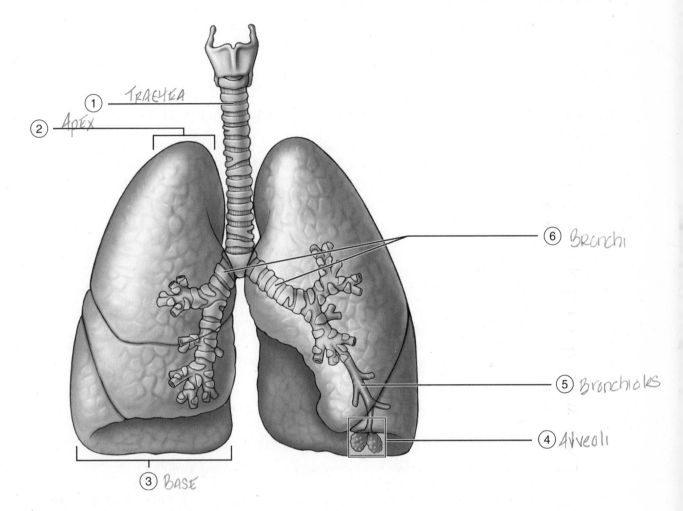

1. ___1___ structure that delivers air to the bronchi
2. ___4___ pulmonary capillaries partially surround these grapelike structures
3. ___5___ structure that delivers oxygen to the alveoli
4. ___4___ lung structure concerned with the exchange of O_2 and CO_2
5. ___2___ apex of the lung
6. ___6___ trachea branches into these large structures
7. ___3___ base of the lung
8. ___4___ grapelike structures that contain surfactants
9. ___1___ windpipe; kept open by rings of cartilage
10. ___6___ large tubes that deliver air to the bronchioles

COLORING

Directions. Color the appropriate areas on the illustration on the previous page.

1. Color the right lung ***purple.***
2. Color the left lung ***blue.***
3. Color the conducting airways ***light brown.***
4. Color the alveoli ***green.***

MATCHING

Thoracic Cavity, Pleural Cavity, and Mediastinum

Directions. Match the following terms to the most appropriate definition by writing the correct letter in the space provided. Some terms may be used more than once. See text pp. 377-384.

A. intrapleural space
B. visceral pleura
C. diaphragm

D. phrenic
E. mediastinum

F. thoracic cavity
G. intercostals

1. __B__ membrane on the outer surface of each lung

2. __A__ space between the visceral and parietal pleural membranes; also called a *potential space*

3. __C__ muscle that separates the thoracic cavity from the abdominal cavity

4. __E__ area between the two lungs; contains other thoracic structures such as the heart, large blood vessels, and the trachea

5. __C__ dome-shaped muscle that is the chief muscle of inhalation

6. __A__ for the lungs to remain expanded, the pressure must be negative within this area

7. __F__ contains the pleural cavity, pericardial cavity, and mediastinum

8. __G__ skeletal muscles between the ribs; they move the rib cage up and out during inhalation

9. __A__ a pneumothorax occurs when air enters this area

10. __D__ motor nerve that stimulates the diaphragm

Student Name _____

MATCHING

Pulmonary Volumes and Capacities

Directions. Match the following terms to the most appropriate definition by writing the correct letter in the space provided. Some terms may be used more than once. See text pp. 387-388.

A. residual volume
B. tidal volume
C. spirometer

D. vital capacity
E. dead air

F. expiratory reserve volume
G. inspiratory reserve volume

1. ___D___ a combination of tidal volume, inspiratory reserve volume, and expiratory reserve volume; about 4600 ml

2. ___A___ the amount of air that remains in the lungs after the exhalation of the expiratory reserve volume; about 1200 ml; this air cannot be exhaled

3. ___C___ an instrument that measures pulmonary volumes

4. ___B___ the amount of air moved into or out of the lungs with each breath; the average is 500 ml

5. ___G___ the amount of air you can inhale after a normal inhalation; about 3000 ml

6. ___D___ a pulmonary capacity that is the maximal amount of air exhaled following maximal inhalation

7. ___F___ the additional volume of air you can exhale after a normal exhalation

8. ___B___ the volume of air you move during normal quiet breathing

9. ___E___ the air that remains in the conducting spaces of the respiratory tract (trachea, bronchi, and bronchioles); it is unavailable for exchange (about 150 ml)

10. ___D___ the following are instructions for its use: "Take the deepest breath possible. Exhale all the air you possibly can into this tube."

ORDERING

Ventilation (Inhalation and Exhalation)

Directions. Place in order the events that occur during one ventilatory cycle (inhalation and exhalation) by writing the correct phrase in the space provided. Two of the steps are given. See text pp. 381-385.

1. The inspiratory neurons in the brain fire action potentials (nerve impulses).
2. Pressure within the lungs (intrapulmonic pressure) decreases.
3. The nerve impulses travel along the phrenic and intercostal nerves to the diaphragm and the intercostal muscles.
4. The diaphragm and the intercostal muscles relax.
5. Air leaves the lungs (air is exhaled).
6. Thoracic volume decreases.
7. The pressure within the lungs (intrapulmonic pressure) increases.
8. The diaphragm and the intercostal muscles contract, thereby enlarging the thoracic cavity.
9. Air moves into the lungs (air is inhaled).
10. The phrenic and intercostal nerves stop firing.

1. The inspiratory neurons in the brain fire action potentials (nerve impulses).
2. ___3_____
3. ___8_____
4. ___2_____
5. Air moves into the lungs (air is inhaled).
6. ___10_____
7. ___4_____
8. ___6_____
9. ___7_____
10. ___5_____

PART II: PUTTING IT ALL TOGETHER

MULTIPLE CHOICE

Directions. Choose the correct answer.

1. Which of the following is least descriptive of the alveoli?

    a. grapelike sacs located very close to the pulmonary capillaries
    b. primarily concerned with gas exchange
    c. located within the lungs
    (d.) contain smooth muscle

2. Bronchi, bronchioles, and alveoli

    a. have rings of cartilage surrounding them.
    b. are sites of gas exchange.
    c. are composed entirely of smooth muscle.
    (d.) are all located within the lungs.

Student Name _____

3. The epiglottis

   a. prevents food and water from entering the respiratory passages.
   b. secretes surfactants.
   c. is considered a true vocal cord.
   d. is concerned with exchange of the respiratory gases.

4. Which of the following refers to the amount of air maximally exhaled following maximal inhalation?

   a. tidal volume
   b. total lung capacity
   c. expiratory reserve volume
   d. vital capacity

5. The trachea does not collapse because it is

   a. located within the lungs.
   b. composed of smooth muscle.
   c. surrounded by ribs.
   d. composed of tough cartilaginous rings.

6. In the absence of surfactants

   a. it is difficult to open the alveoli.
   b. bronchioles relax.
   c. the alveoli fill with water.
   d. air enters the intrapleural space.

7. What is the effect of contraction of the diaphragm and the intercostal muscles?

   a. increases the volume of the thoracic cavity
   b. forces air out of the lungs
   c. closes the epiglottis
   d. stimulates the secretion of pulmonary surfactants

8. The phrenic nerve

   a. causes swallowing.
   b. supplies the epiglottis so that food is diverted to the esophagus.
   c. stimulates the diaphragm to contract.
   d. exits from the spinal cord at the L3 level.

9. Which transport mechanism causes the respiratory gases to move across the alveolar-pulmonary capillary membrane?

   a. filtration
   b. osmosis
   c. diffusion
   d. active transport pump

10. Why does a stab wound to the chest cause the lung to collapse?

   a. Infection develops within the intrapleural space.
   b. The intrapleural pressure increases.
   c. Pressure within the lung increases.
   d. Bleeding causes hypotension and septic shock.

11. What does Boyle's law state?

   a. when volume increases, pressure increases
   b. when volume decreases, pressure decreases
   c. when volume increases, pressure decreases
   d. change in volume has no effect on pressure

12. How is most oxygen transported in the blood?

   a. by hemoglobin
   b. as bicarbonate
   c. by pulmonary surfactants
   d. dissolved in plasma

13. How is most carbon dioxide transported in the blood?

   a. by hemoglobin
   b. as bicarbonate
   c. by pulmonary surfactants
   d. dissolved in plasma

14. The medullary respiratory control center

   a. is located in the cerebrum.
   b. is sensitive to the depressant effects of opioids (narcotics).
   c. can increase respiratory rate but cannot decrease respiratory rate.
   d. can decrease respiratory rate but cannot increase respiratory rate.

15. An increase in blood _____ is most likely to increase the rate of breathing.

   a. volume
   b. CO_2
   c. bilirubin
   d. calcium

16. What is the consequence of a severed spinal cord at the level of C2?

    a. quadriplegia with no respiratory impairment
    b. hemiplegia with no respiratory involvement
    c. quadriplegia and respiratory paralysis
    d. paraplegia with no respiratory involvement

17. Who has a dome-shaped belly?

    a. Al V. Oli
    b. Tray Kea
    c. Di A. Phragm
    d. Hy Poxia

18. Which of the following statements is true about the aging respiratory system?

    a. By age 70, vital capacity has decreased about 33%.
    b. Aging is associated with a decrease in vital capacity but with an increase in the total number of alveoli.
    c. By age 70, all of the alveoli have collapsed and gas exchange is occurring across the walls of the bronchioles.
    d. Because of the decrease in vital capacity, a person older than 70 years should not exercise.

CASE STUDY

T.K. went to the doctor's office complaining of extreme fatigue, shortness of breath, fever, and a persistent cough of 3 weeks' duration. An x-ray revealed left lower lobar pneumonia with areas of alveolar collapse (atelectasis). He was given a prescription for an antibiotic.

1. What is the effect of left lower lobar pneumonia and atelectasis on breathing?

    a. There are fewer alveoli available for gas exchange.
    b. Rapid, shallow breathing can easily compensate for the collapsed alveoli; no further treatment is required.
    c. The alveoli in the left lower lobe can function fairly well if they fill with blood from the pulmonary capillaries.
    d. There will be no effect on breathing and Po_2.

2. Which of the following is the underlying cause of the fever?

    a. atelectasis
    b. infection
    c. cyanosis
    d. hypoxia

3. Coughing

    a. is the body's attempt to clear the respiratory passages.
    b. should be completely suppressed to rest the lungs.
    c. should be suppressed because it may spread the infection to the unaffected lung.
    d. should be suppressed because it impairs the effectiveness of the antibiotics.

Student Name _____

PART III: CHALLENGE YOURSELF

GROUPS AND PUZZLE

1. Which group is incorrect?

    a. structures of the bronchial tree: bronchi, bronchioles, alveoli
    b. "breathing" nerves: phrenic, intercostals, cauda equina
    c. paranasal sinuses: frontal, maxillary, sphenoidal, ethmoidal
    d. parts of the pharynx: oropharynx, nasopharynx, laryngopharynx

2. Which group is incorrect?

    a. pulmonary volumes: tidal volume, inspiratory reserve volume, expiratory reserve volume
    b. paranasal sinuses: frontal, maxillary, sphenoidal, ethmoidal
    c. structures of the upper respiratory tract: trachea, pharynx, larynx, bronchioles
    d. respiratory gases: oxygen, carbon dioxide

3. Which group is incorrect?

    a. pulmonary volumes: tidal volume, vital capacity
    b. "breathing" nerves: phrenic, intercostals
    c. paranasal sinuses: frontal, maxillary, sphenoidal, ethmoidal
    d. structures of the upper respiratory tract: trachea, pharynx, larynx

PUZZLE

Hint: Sneeze and Wheeze

Directions. Perform the following functions on the Sequence of Words below. When all the functions have been performed, you are left with word(s) that are related to the hint. Record your answer below.

Functions: remove the following

1. the structures that are called the *throat, voicebox,* and *windpipe*
2. the terms that describe the breathing in and breathing out phases of ventilation (4)
3. the respiratory gases (2)
4. serous membranes (2) located within the thoracic cavity
5. maximal exhalation following maximal inhalation
6. grapelike respiratory structure concerned with the exchange of O_2 and CO_2
7. when volume increases, pressure decreases
8. primary muscle of inhalation and its motor nerve
9. amount of air moved during normal quiet breathing
10. a color-consequence of hypoxemia

Sequence of Words

ALVEOLUSCYANOSISBRONCHOCONSTRICTIONINSPIRATIONDIAPHRAGMVITALCAP
ACITYCARBONDIOXIDEVISCERALPLEURATRACHEAEXHALATIONPHRENICBOYLE'SL
AWALLERGYOXYGENPHARYNXLARYNXINHALATIONTIDALVOLUMEPARIETALPLEURA
HISTAMINEEXPIRATION

Answer: _____, _____, _____

BODY TOON

Hint: What does this view have to do with a runny nose?

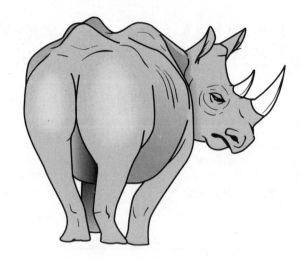

Answer: Both are called rhino-rear (rhinorrhea).

23

Digestive System

Objectives

1. List four functions of the digestive system.

2. Describe the four layers of the digestive tract.

3. Describe the structure and functions of the organs of the digestive tract.

4. Describe the structure and functions of the accessory organs of the digestive tract.

5. Explain the physiology of digestion and absorption.

6. Describe the effects of amylases, proteases, and lipases.

7. Describe the role of bile in the digestion of fats.

8. Describe five categories of nutrients.

PART I: MASTERING THE BASICS

MATCHING

Terms Related to the Digestive System

Directions. Match the following terms to the most appropriate definition by writing the correct letter in the space provided. See text pp. 396-400.

A. alimentary canal   D. chemical digestion   F. absorption
B. digestion   E. bolus   G. mechanical digestion
C. peristalsis

1. __F__ process by which the end-products of digestion move across the walls of the alimentary canal into the blood
2. __A__ the hollow tube that extends from the mouth to the anus
3. __B__ process by which food is broken down into simpler substances that can be absorbed
4. __G__ type of digestion that physically breaks food into smaller pieces
5. __C__ a rhythmic contraction of the muscles of the digestive tract that moves food forward toward the anus
6. __E__ ball-like mass of food that is mixed with saliva in the mouth; it is swallowed and turned into chyme in the stomach
7. __D__ type of digestion accomplished by the digestive enzymes
8. __A__ also called the *digestive tract* or the *gastrointestinal (GI) tract*
9. __G__ type of digestion that includes the chewing and mashing of food

MATCHING

Teeth and Related Structures

Directions. Match the following terms to the most appropriate definition by writing the correct letter in the space provided. See text pp. 398-400.

A. deciduous   E. pulp   H. root canal
B. permanent   F. dentin   I. cementum
C. crown   G. root   J. enamel
D. gingiva

1. __A__ term for the 20 baby (milk) teeth
2. __G__ part of the tooth embedded within the jawbone
3. __C__ part of the tooth above the level of the gum
4. __I__ part of the tooth that anchors the root to the periodontal membrane; it holds the tooth in place
5. __E__ part of the tooth containing the nerves, blood vessels, and connective tissue; it supplies the tooth with sensation and nutrients

6. __D__ term for the gum

7. __J__ hard, brittle covering of the crown of the tooth

8. __F__ bonelike material that makes up the bulk of the tooth

9. __B__ these 32 teeth replace the baby teeth

10. __H__ the extension of the pulp cavity into the root

MATCHING

Digestive Enzymes, Hormones, and Other Secretions

Directions. Match the following terms to the most appropriate definition by writing the correct letter in the space provided. Some terms may be used more than once. See text pp. 410-417.

A. amylase(s)   F. cholecystokinin   K. gastric juice

B. lipases   G. hydrochloric acid   L. saliva

C. bile   H. chyle   M. disaccharidases

D. chyme   I. secretin

E. intrinsic factor   J. proteases

1. __L__ secretion of the salivary glands; contains water, electrolytes, mucus, and ptyalin

2. __D__ partially digested food that is mashed into a pastelike consistency in the stomach

3. __E__ a deficiency of this substance leads to pernicious anemia

4. __G__ a substance that is secreted by the parietal cells of the stomach; it lowers the gastric pH

5. __C__ a substance produced by the liver and stored in the gallbladder

6. __A__ enzyme found in saliva; also called *ptyalin*

7. __J__ classification of pepsin, trypsin, chymotrypsin, and enterokinase

8. __M__ sucrase, maltase, lactase

9. __H__ milky-white lymph caused by fat digestion

10. __J__ enzymes that digest proteins to small peptides and amino acids

11. __B__ enzymes that digest fats to fatty acids and glycerol

12. __E__ a substance secreted by the parietal cells of the stomach; it is necessary for the absorption of vitamin B_{12}

13. __I__ a hormone secreted by the walls of the duodenum; it stimulates the pancreas to secrete a bicarbonate-rich substance

14. __A__ enzymes that digest carbohydrates to disaccharides

15. __F__ a hormone secreted by the walls of the duodenum; it stimulates the pancreas to secrete an enzyme-rich substance

16. __K__ secretion of the glands of the stomach; it contains HCl, intrinsic factor, water, electrolytes, and digestive enzymes

17. __F__ a hormone secreted by the walls of the duodenum; it causes the gallbladder to contract and to eject bile into the common bile duct

18. __C__ an emulsifying agent

MATCHING

Parts of the Digestive Tract

Directions. Match the following terms to the most appropriate definition by writing the correct letter in the space provided. Some terms may be used more than once. See text pp. 398-414.

A. stomach
B. small intestine
C. pancreas
D. liver

E. gallbladder
F. buccal cavity
G. salivary glands

H. esophagus
I. epiglottis
J. large intestine

1. ___D___ organ that produces bile and secretes it into the hepatic bile ducts
2. ___I___ structure that directs food and water away from the larynx into the esophagus
3. ___H___ the "food tube;" it carries food from the pharynx to the stomach
4. ___B___ the common bile duct empties bile into this structure
5. ___E___ pear-shaped sac that attaches to the underside of the liver; it concentrates and stores bile
6. ___A___ the parietal cells of this organ secrete hydrochloric acid and intrinsic factor
7. ___E___ organ that is connected to the common bile duct by the cystic duct
8. ___G___ parotid, sublingual, and submandibular
9. ___A___ organ that is divided into the fundus, body, and pylorus
10. ___B___ most digestion and absorption occur within this structure
11. ___A___ the primary function of this organ is to deliver chyme to the duodenum at the proper rate
12. ___A___ the walls of this organ are thrown into folds called *rugae*
13. ___J___ divisions include the cecum, colon, rectum, and anal canal
14. ___C___ organ that secretes the most potent digestive enzymes
15. ___G___ an inflammation of one of these structures is called *mumps*
16. ___A___ organ that contains mucus cells, parietal cells, and chief cells
17. ___B___ the inner lining of this structure is characterized by villi and microvilli; brush border cells
18. ___B___ divisions include the duodenum, jejunum, and ileum
19. ___A___ landmarks of this organ include the greater curvature and lesser curvature
20. ___J___ this structure has bends or curves called the *hepatic flexure* and the *splenic flexure*
21. ___B___ the walls of this structure secrete cholecystokinin
22. ___J___ a colostomy is a surgical procedure performed on this structure
23. ___J___ the appendix is attached to this structure
24. ___B___ the walls of this structure secrete the disaccharidases
25. ___F___ part of the mouth or oral cavity
26. ___B___ the pylorus connects the stomach with this structure
27. ___J___ flatus, feces, and defecation are most related to this structure
28. ___D___ the chief organ of drug detoxification
29. ___C___ organ that secretes insulin, glucagon, trypsin, and a bicarbonate-rich secretion
30. ___B___ peristalsis is pendulum-like (sways back and forth) in this organ

Student Name _____

READ THE DIAGRAM

Directions. Fill in the blanks with the numbers on the diagram. See text pp. 398-414.

1. __12__ organ that produces bile and secretes it into the hepatic bile ducts

2. __6__ the walls of this structure secrete cholecystokinin

3. __3__ "food tube" that carries food from the pharynx to the stomach

4. __5__ pear-shaped sac that attaches to the underside of the liver; it concentrates and stores bile

5. __4__ parietal cells of this organ that secrete hydrochloric acid and intrinsic factor

6. __11__ parotid, sublingual, and submandibular

7. __4__ organ that is divided into the fundus, body, and pylorus

8. __6__ most digestion and absorption occur within this structure

9. __4__ the primary function of this organ is to deliver chyme to the duodenum at the proper rate

10. __4__ the walls of this organ are thrown into folds called *rugae*

11. __7__ divisions include the cecum, colon, rectum, and anal canal

12. __10__ the organ that secretes the most potent digestive enzymes

13. __11__ an inflammation of one of these structures is called *mumps*

14. __4__ this organ contains mucus cells, parietal cells, and chief cells

15. __6__ the inner lining of this structure is characterized by villi and microvilli; brush border cells

16. __6__ divisions include the duodenum, jejunum, and ileum

17. __4__ landmarks of this organ include the greater curvature and lesser curvature

18. __7__ this structure has bends or curves called the *hepatic flexure* and the *splenic flexure*

19. __6__ the pylorus connects the stomach with this structure

20. __7__ flatus, feces, and defecation are most related to this structure

21. __12__ the chief organ of drug detoxification

22. __10__ this organ secretes insulin, glucagon, trypsin, and a bicarbonate-rich secretion

23. __6__ peristalsis is pendulum-like (sways back and forth) in this organ

DRAWING AND COLORING

Directions. Using the illustration on the previous page, perform the following exercises.

1. Draw a circle around the LES.
2. Place an X over the fundus of the stomach.
3. Draw an arrow to the pylorus.
4. Draw rugae in the stomach wall.
5. Draw an ulcer on the greater curvature of the stomach.
6. Write the word HEPATIC over the proper structure.
7. Draw some stones in the gallbladder.
8. Place a Y at the point where the common bile duct empties into the small intestine.
9. Place a Z over the area of the appendix.
10. Color the biliary tree green.
11. Color the alimentary canal light blue.

ORDERING

Directions. A piece of food starts in the mouth. Trace the movement of the food from the mouth to the anus (use the words listed below). See text pp. 398-409, 416.

jejunum	duodenum	descending colon
pharynx	rectum	stomach
esophagus	ascending colon	ileum
transverse colon	hepatic flexure	cecum
LES	ileocecal valve	anus
sigmoid colon		

1. Mouth
2. pharynx
3. esophagus
4. LES
5. Stomach
6. pyloric sphincter
7. duodenum
8. jejunum
9. ileum
10. ileocecal valve

11. cecum
12. ascending colon
13. hepatic flexure
14. transverse colon
15. splenic flexure
16. descending colon
17. sigmoid
18. rectum
19. anus

Student Name _____

READ THE DIAGRAM

Directions. Referring to the diagram (Figure 23-11) in the textbook, fill in the blanks with the letter of the column or the appropriate words. See text pp. 414-417.

1. __B__ the column that shows the end-products of protein digestion
2. __Bile__ hepatic secretion that emulsifies fat globules into tiny fat globules
3. __A__ the column that makes glucose, fructose, and galactose
4. __→__ enzymes that break down carbohydrates into disaccharides *Amylases*
5. __→__ result of disaccharide digestion *Monosaccharides*
6. __→__ result of trypsin, chymotrypsin, pepsin, and enterokinase digestion *AminoAcids*
7. __→__ digestion of this substance yields amino acids *Proteins*
8. __→__ digestion of this substance yields sucrose, maltose, and lactose *Polysaccharides*
9. __Lipase__ enzyme that digests fats to fatty acids and glycerol
10. __Bile__ an emulsifying agent
11. __A__ column that illustrates the digestion of starch to glucose
12. __A__ column that illustrates the effects of amylases and disaccharidases

MATCHING

Nutrients, Vitamins, and Minerals

Directions. Match the following terms to the most appropriate definition by writing the correct letter in the space provided. See text pp. 417-418.

A. essential amino acids
B. nonessential amino acids
C. linoleic acid
D. cellulose

E. glucose
F. complete protein
G. incomplete protein
H. saturated fats

I. unsaturated fats
J. vitamins
K. minerals

1. __E__ simplest carbohydrate that is the major fuel used to make ATP
2. __G__ protein that does not contain all of the essential amino acids; these include the vegetable proteins such as nuts, grains, and legumes
3. __B__ amino acids that can be synthesized by the body and do not have to be consumed in the diet
4. __H__ a fat that is solid at room temperature; examples include butter and lard
5. __J__ small, organic molecules that help regulate cell metabolism; classified as water-soluble and fat-soluble
6. __D__ complex carbohydrate found primarily in vegetables; it provides dietary fiber and bulk to the stools
7. __K__ inorganic substances necessary for normal body function
8. __I__ fat that is liquid at room temperature; usually called *oil*
9. __A__ amino acids that cannot be synthesized by the body and must therefore be consumed in the diet
10. __C__ essential fatty acid that is a necessary part of the cell membrane
11. __F__ a protein that contains all of the essential amino acids; it is found primarily in animal sources such as meat and in some grains and legumes

MATCHING

Vitamins and Minerals

Directions. Match the following terms to the most appropriate definition by writing the correct letter in the space provided. Some terms may be used more than once. See text pp. 418-419.

A.   water-soluble vitamins   E.   calcium   I.   fat-soluble vitamins

B.   vitamin A   F.   iodine   J.   sodium

C.   vitamin K   G.   vitamin C   K.   vitamin B group

D.   iron   H.   vitamin D

1.   _I_   classification of vitamins A, D, E, K

2.   _H_   vitamin necessary for the absorption of calcium and for the development of strong bones

3.   _B_   a vitamin deficiency that causes night blindness

4.   _H_   a vitamin deficiency that causes rickets or soft bones (osteomalacia)

5.   _G_   a vitamin deficiency that causes scurvy, a disease characterized by skin lesions and an inability to heal injured tissue

6.   _J_   mineral that helps regulate extracellular volume (including blood volume)

7.   _A_   classification of vitamins B and C

8.   _E_   mineral necessary for bone growth

9.   _F_   mineral necessary for the synthesis of thyroid hormone, which in turn regulates metabolic rate

10. _D_   mineral necessary for the synthesis of hemoglobin and the transport of oxygen

11. _C_   vitamin necessary for the synthesis of prothrombin, a clotting factor

12. _K_   vitamins such as thiamine, niacin, and pyridoxine

13. _C_   deficiency of this vitamin causes bleeding

PART II: PUTTING IT ALL TOGETHER

MULTIPLE CHOICE

Directions. Choose the correct answer.

1.   Chyme is
     a.   delivered to the duodenum by the stomach.
     b.   found in the lacteals.
     c.   a pastelike mixture that is stored in the gallbladder.
     d.   formed in the mouth in response to ptyalin.

2.   The mesentery, omentum, and peritoneal membranes
     a.   are located within the alimentary canal.
     b.   secrete mucus.
     c.   secrete digestive enzymes.
     d.   are serous membranes located within the abdominal cavity.

Student Name _____

3. Bile is

   a. synthesized by the gallbladder and stored in the liver.
   b. classified as a lipase.
   c. synthesized by the pancreas and stored in the gallbladder.
   d. stored by the gallbladder and released in response to CCK.

4. What is the reason that medications are absorbed rapidly when administered sublingually (under the tongue)?

   a. Acid in the saliva dissolves the drugs rapidly.
   b. Ptyalin secreted by the salivary glands digests the drugs, making them more absorbable.
   c. The rich supply of blood vessels under the tongue absorbs the drug.
   d. The warmth of the tongue dissolves the drugs quickly.

5. Which structure does not "see" bile?

   a. hepatic duct
   b. ampulla of Vater
   c. portal vein
   d. cystic duct

6. What nervous statement is true about the GI tract?

   a. the pudendal nerve innervates the descending colon and sigmoid
   b. parasympathetic nerve stimulation decreases peristalsis and decreases secretions
   c. vagal nerve stimulation decreases peristalsis and decreases secretions
   d. blockade of vagal activity slows peristalsis and decreases GI secretions

7. The esophagus enters the abdominal cavity through an opening in the diaphragm. What might happen if the opening is too wide?

   a. The heart will fall into the abdominal cavity.
   b. The stomach may herniate or slide up into the chest cavity.
   c. The person will not be able to swallow.
   d. Hydrochloric acid will fill the chest cavity.

8. Occasionally in infancy, the pylorus is too narrow and hampers the movement of chyme from the stomach into the duodenum. This condition is most likely to cause which symptom?

   a. projectile vomiting
   b. cyanosis
   c. jaundice
   d. diarrhea

9. Which of the following is not true of the biliary tree?

   a. includes the hepatic ducts, cystic duct, and the common bile duct
   b. carries bile
   c. empties bile into the portal vein
   d. "connects" the liver, gallbladder, and duodenum

10. An amylase

   a. digests fats.
   b. emulsifies fat.
   c. digests carbohydrates.
   d. assembles amino acids into small peptides.

11. If the peristalsis in the large intestine slows

   a. all waste will be absorbed across the colon wall into the hepatic portal system.
   b. water absorption across the wall of the colon increases, thereby causing a dry or constipated stool.
   c. the person develops diarrhea.
   d. bile refluxes into the main pancreatic duct.

12. What is the primary function of the large intestine?

   a. secretion of potent digestive enzymes
   b. absorption of water and some electrolytes
   c. absorption of the end-products of digestion
   d. secretion of cholecystokinin

13. Cholecystokinin

   a. is secreted by the pancreas.
   b. is secreted in response to the presence of fat in the duodenum.
   c. causes the liver to synthesize lipase.
   d. is a lipase.

14. Which of the following is most likely to result in peritonitis?

    a. GERD
    b. cholecystitis
    c. ruptured appendix
    d. pyloric stenosis

15. Peristalsis

    a. occurs only within the stomach and small intestine.
    b. is the same as mastication.
    c. only occurs following deglutition.
    d. moves food along the digestive tract.

16. A paralytic ileus is

    a. a deficiency of digestive enzymes resulting in malabsorption.
    b. a cessation of peristalsis.
    c. a consequence of hyperacidity.
    d. a major cause of peritonitis.

17. Since hepatic function declines with age, which statement describes an older adult?

    a. likely to be jaundiced
    b. should not eat fat
    c. may require a smaller dosage of a drug
    d. should consume no alcohol

18. The ampulla of Vater and the sphincter of Oddi

    a. are at the base of the common bile duct.
    b. control the entrance of chyme into the pylorus.
    c. are part of the LES.
    d. are valvelike structures within the hepatic portal circulation.

19. Who is most likely to drool?

    a. Sue Crose
    b. Sal I. Vary
    c. Amy Lase
    d. Chyle

CASE STUDY

A.B., a 65-year-old retired nurse, had no previous history of major illness. Following a meal of fried chicken and gravy, she complained of moderate to severe midepigastric pain that radiated to the right subscapular region. She became nauseated and vomited. Since there was no improvement in either the pain or nausea, she called her physician the following morning. The physician noticed that she was jaundiced and that her stools had become clay-colored. She was diagnosed with cholecystitis (inflammation of the gallbladder) and choledocholithiasis (stones in the common bile duct). She was scheduled for a cholecystectomy (surgical removal of the gallbladder) on the following day. One of the preoperative laboratory tests (prothrombin time) indicated that she was hypoprothrombinemic; she was therefore given an intramuscular injection of vitamin K.

1. Which of the following best indicates the reason that the fried chicken and gravy stimulated the gallbladder attack?

    a. Fat irritates the gastric lining, causing an excess secretion of hydrochloric acid.
    b. Fat relaxes the lower esophageal sphincter, causing heartburn.
    c. The presence of fat in the duodenum stimulates the inflamed gallbladder to contract.
    d. The cholesterol in the fats causes stone formation.

2. What causes the jaundice to develop?

    a. There is a hypersecretion of digestive enzymes.
    b. The inflamed gallbladder causes hemolysis.
    c. The inflamed gallbladder secretes a poison that destroys the liver.
    d. The stones block the flow of bile through the common bile duct.

3. What substance is responsible for the jaundice?

    a. amylase
    b. lipase
    c. hydrochloric acid
    d. bilirubin

Student Name _____

4. Why was she hypoprothrombinemic?

    a. The lack of bile in the duodenum decreased the absorption of vitamin K, a factor necessary for the synthesis of prothrombin.
    b. The vomiting caused a vitamin K deficiency; vitamin K is necessary for the synthesis of several clotting factors.
    c. The stones injured the common bile duct, causing it to bleed and depleting the body of clotting factors such as prothrombin.
    d. Prothrombin is synthesized by the gallbladder, so its production decreases because of the inflammation.

5. What is the most likely consequence of hypoprothrombinemia?

    a. jaundice
    b. hypertension
    c. bleeding
    d. hemolysis

6. Vitamin K was given in order to

    a. stimulate the hepatic synthesis of prothrombin
    b. dissolve the stones
    c. stimulate the kidneys to excrete the excess bilirubin
    d. relieve the pain

7. Why had her stools become clay-colored?

    a. Undigested fat in the duodenum makes the stools appear light.
    b. Because the stones had blocked the common bile duct, there was a decreased amount of bile pigment in the stool.
    c. Excess bile in the duodenum makes the stools appear light.
    d. Small, gray stones washed into the stool from the common bile duct, thereby changing its color.

PART III: CHALLENGE YOURSELF!

GROUPS AND PUZZLE

1. Which group is incorrect?

    a. salivary glands: sublingual, submandibular, parotid
    b. small intestine: duodenum, jejunum, ileum
    c. digestive enzymes: amylase, protease, lipase
    d. hormones: gastrin, bile, cholecystokinin

2. Which group is incorrect?

    a. parts of the stomach: pylorus, fundus, body
    b. hormones: gastrin, secretin, cholecystokinin
    c. disaccharidases: maltase, lipase, sucrase
    d. biliary tree structures: cystic duct, hepatic ducts, common bile duct

3. Which group is incorrect?

    a. small intestine: duodenum, jejunum, ileum
    b. cells in the stomach: chief, parietal, mucus-secreting
    c. blood vessels of the portal system: portal vein, superior mesenteric vein, splenic vein
    d. peritoneal membranes: mesentery, omentum, villus

PUZZLE

Hint: Bile Aisle and Main Vein

Directions. Perform the following functions on the Sequence of Words below. When all the functions have been performed, you are left with word(s) that are related to the hint. Record your answer below.

Functions: remove the following

1. the three parts of the small intestine
2. the appendix attaches to this structure
3. the distal end of the stomach
4. organ that secretes the most potent digestive enzymes
5. the circular muscle at the distal esophagus
6. food tube
7. valve that separates the small intestine from the large intestine
8. organ that secretes bile
9. organ that stores bile
10. four parts of the colon
11. sphincter at the distal common bile duct
12. major parasympathetic nerve supplying the gut
13. disaccharidases
14. a major pancreatic protease
15. enzyme that digests fats

Sequence of Words

JEJUNUMGALLBLADDERTRANSVERSELOWERESOPHAGEALSPHINCTERASCENDINGC
OMMONBILEDUCTCECUMLIPASEPANCREASLACTASEESOPHAGUSSUCRASEPYLORUSV
AGUSDESCENDINGDUODENUMSIGMOIDPORTALVEINLIVERILIUMILEOCECALVALVEMA
LTASEODDITRYPSIN

Answer: <u>Common Bile Duct, portal vein</u>

Student Name _____

BODY TOONS

Hint: A perfect ending to the story of digestion

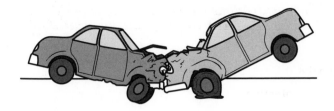

Hint: Two punctuation marks

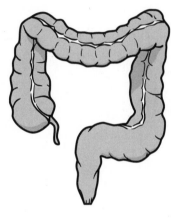 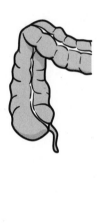

24

Urinary System

Answer Key: Textbook page references are provided as a guide for answering these questions. A complete answer key was provided for your instructor.

Objectives

1. List four organs of excretion.

2. Describe the major organs of the urinary system.

3. Describe the location, structure, blood supply, nerve supply, and functions of the kidneys.

4. Explain the role of the nephron unit in the formation of urine.

5. Explain the three processes involved in the formation of urine: filtration, reabsorption, and secretion.

6. Describe the hormonal control of water and electrolytes by the kidneys.

7. List the normal constituents of urine.

8. Describe the structure and function of the ureters, urinary bladder, and urethra.

PART I: MASTERING THE BASICS

MATCHING

The Urinary System

Directions. Match the following terms to the most appropriate definition by writing the correct letter in the space provided. Some words may be used more than once. See text pp. 426-428.

A. ureters

B. kidneys

C. hilus

D. renal pelvis

E. bladder

F. renal pyramids

G. renal capsule

H. urethra

I. renal columns

J. calyces

1. __A__ tubes that conduct urine from the kidneys to the bladder

2. __H__ tube that conducts urine from the bladder to the exterior for elimination

3. __E__ reservoir that receives and stores urine

4. __E__ a Foley catheter is inserted into this organ for drainage

5. __B__ bean-shaped organs that make urine

6. __A__ pathogens can ascend from the bladder through these tubes to the kidneys, thereby causing a kidney infection

7. __E__ structure that is involved in urinary retention

8. __E__ structure that contains the trigone, a triangle formed by the two points of entrance of the ureters and the exit point of the urethra

9. __H__ the external sphincter surrounds the upper region of this structure

10. __E__ the internal sphincter is located at the exit of this structure

11. __H__ the prostate gland encircles the proximal end of this structure

12. __C__ the indentation of the bean-shaped kidney; it is the point where blood vessels, nerves, and the ureter enter or exit the kidney

13. __E__ the wall of this structure is arranged in rugae to allow for expansion

14. __D__ basin within the kidney that collects the urine made by the kidney

15. __I__ the lighter, outer region of the kidney, called the *renal cortex*, extends inward to form these structures

16. __F__ the darker, inner region of the kidney, called the *renal medulla*, forms these striped cone-shaped regions

17. __J__ cuplike edges of the renal pelvis that receive the urine from the renal pyramids and empty it into the renal pelvis

18. __G__ tough outer lining that encases the kidney

19. __E__ storage structure that empties during micturition

20. __E__ storage structure that contains the detrusor muscle

Na$^+$ = Sodium
K$^+$ = Potassium

Student Name _____

READ THE DIAGRAM

Urinary System

Directions. Referring to the illustration, indicate the parts of the urinary system by writing the correct numbers on the lines provided. See text pp. 426-428, 436-439.

1. __2__ tubes that conduct urine from the kidneys to the bladder

2. __1__ urine-making organs

3. __8__ reservoir that stores urine

4. __8__ a Foley catheter drains urine from this organ

5. __2__ pathogens can ascend from the bladder through this tube to the kidney, thereby causing a kidney infection

6. __3__ detrusor muscle

7. __7__ prostate gland encircles the proximal end of this structure

8. __5__ a triangle formed by the two points of entrance of the ureters and the exit point of the urethra

9. __6__ sphincter at the base of the bladder

10. __4__ the ureter enters the bladder at this point

11. __2__ a stone in this structure causes urine to back up into the kidney

12. __8__ cystitis is an infection of this organ

13. __8__ the organ that contracts, causing micturition

14. __8__ the organ of concern with urinary retention

15. __1__ the organ of concern with renal suppression

① Kidney
② Ureter
③ Detrusor Muscle
④ Urethral Opening
⑤ Trigone
⑥ Internal
⑦ Urethra
⑧ Bladder

MATCHING

Nephron Unit

Directions. Match the following terms to the most appropriate definition by writing the correct letter in the space provided. Some terms may be used more than once. See text pp. 428-434.

A. peritubular capillaries	C. proximal convoluted tubule	E. distal convoluted tubule
B. loop of Henle	D. collecting duct	F. glomerulus (glomeruli)

1. ___F___   tuft of capillaries across which water and solute are filtered

2. ___D___   the distal convoluted tubule empties urine into this structure

3. ___D___   structure that is most concerned with the concentration of urine

4. ___A___   vascular structure that surrounds the tubules; involved in reabsorption and secretion

5. ___A___   the efferent arteriole extends and becomes this structure

6. ___C___   most reabsorption occurs across the walls of this tubular structure

7. ___D___   the site at which ADH is most active

8. ___F___   the afferent and efferent arterioles bracket (form bookends to) this structure

9. ___D___   the final adjustment of urine occurs at this site

10. ___b___   the proximal convoluted tubule extends as this structure

11. ___E___   site at which aldosterone is most active

12. ___F___   these capillaries sit within the C-shaped Bowman's capsule

13. ___A___   vascular structure that empties blood into the venules and eventually into the renal vein

14. ___A___   the process of secretion causes solute to move from this structure into the tubules

15. ___b___   composed of an ascending and a descending limb

16. ___A___   reabsorption causes water and solute to move from the tubule into this structure

17. ___b___   hairpin structure between the proximal and distal tubules

18. ___D___   tubular structure that carries urine from the distal tubule to the calyx

Student Name _____

READ THE DIAGRAM

Nephron Unit

LABEL DIAGRAM ONLY (DO NOT ANSWER ? 1-12)

Directions. Referring to the diagram, fill in the blanks with the correct number. Some numbers may be used more than once. See text pp. 428-434.

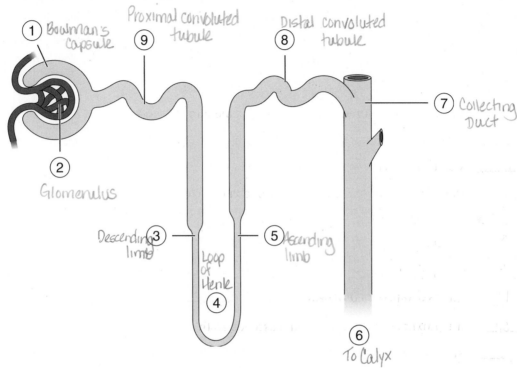

1. _2_   tuft of capillaries across which water and solute are filtered
2. _7_   the distal convoluted tubule empties urine into this structure
3. _7_   structure that is most concerned with the concentration of urine
4. _9_   most reabsorption occurs across the walls of this tubular structure
5. _7_   site at which ADH is most active
6. _8_   site at which aldosterone is most active
7. _2_   the afferent and efferent arterioles "bookend" this structure
8. _7_   the final adjustment of urine occurs at this site
9. _3,4_   the proximal convoluted tubule extends as this structure
10. _1_   the glomerulus sits within this structure
11. _4_   composed of an ascending and descending limb
12. _6_   urine on its way to the calyx

COLORING

Directions. Using the illustration above, color the appropriate areas as indicated below.

1. Color the glomerulus **red.**
2. Color the proximal and distal convoluted tubules **green.**
3. Color the loop of Henle **blue.**
4. Color the collecting duct **yellow.**

ORDERING

The Flow of Urine

Directions. Using the words below, trace the flow of urine from its formation (filtration of water and solute across the glomeruli) to its elimination from the body. See text pp. 428-434.

descending limb (loop of Henle)	ascending limb (loop of Henle)	bladder
	distal convoluted tubule	Bowman's capsule
collecting duct	ureter	proximal convoluted tubule
renal pelvis	calyces	
urethra		

1. filtration of water and solute across the glomeruli
2. bowman's capsule
3. proximal convoluted tubule
4. descending limb (loop of Henle)
5. ascending limb
6. distal convoluted tubule
7. collecting duct
8. calyces
9. renal pelvis
10. ureter
11. bladder
12. urethra

Student Name _____

MATCHING

Hormones and Enzymes

Directions. Match the following terms to the most appropriate definition by writing the correct letter in the space provided. Some terms may be used more than once. See text pp. 431-433.

A. ADH
B. aldosterone
C. renin

D. angiotensin II
E. ANP
F. converting enzyme

G. PTH
H. erythropoietin
I. BNP

1. __D__ hormone that stimulates the adrenal cortex to secrete aldosterone and causes vasoconstriction of the peripheral blood vessels, thereby elevating blood pressure

2. __B__ the adrenal cortical hormone that stimulates the distal tubule to reabsorb sodium and excrete potassium

3. __F__ enzyme that changes angiotensin I to angiotensin II

4. __B__ the mineralocorticoid that is called the *salt-retaining hormone*

5. __A__ secreted by the posterior pituitary gland; this hormone affects the permeability of the collecting duct to water

6. __H__ released by the kidney in response to hypoxemia; it stimulates red blood cell production by the bone marrow

7. __C__ secreted by the juxtaglomerular apparatus (JGA) when blood pressure and/or blood volume decreases

8. __E__ secreted by the atrial walls in response to an increase in blood volume; it causes the excretion of sodium and water

9. __C__ enzyme that activates angiotensinogen to angiotensin I

10. __A__ a deficiency of this hormone causes polyuria (diuresis), sometimes up to 25 liters of urine per day; this hormone deficiency disease is called *diabetes insipidus*

11. __G__ stimulates the renal tubules to reabsorb calcium and to excrete phosphate

12. __I__ hormone that is released in response to ventricular stretch; elevated in heart failure

13. __G__ a deficiency of this hormone causes hypocalcemic tetany

14. __H__ hormone that is deficient in a patient with chronic renal failure: causes anemia

15. __D__ ACE inhibitors block the formation of this vasopressor hormone

16. __B__ a deficiency of this hormone causes the urinary excretion of Na^+ and water and the retention of K^+

17. __G__ an excess of this hormone can cause hypercalcemia and kidney stones

TELL A STORY

Going Up!

Directions. Use the words below, fill in the blanks to complete the story. See text pp. 436-439.

pyelonephritis	dysuria	ascending infection
analgesia	pyuria	hematuria
antimicrobial	cystitis	

Polly Uria is a college freshman who came to the student health office complaining of flank pain, night sweats, fever, and "feeling terrible." She reported that she had been experiencing frequency, urgency, and pain on urination (called _dysuria_____) for one week prior to the onset of fever and pain. She did not seek medical treatment at this time because she was busy with exams. Instead, she had self-medicated with an over-the-counter azo dye preparation. (The azo dye relieved the pain; this effect is called _analgesia____.) The azo dye, however, does not kill the pathogens and therefore does not exert an _antimicrobial_ effect.) A cloudy and foul-smelling urine sample indicated pus and bacteria in the urine (called ___pyuris_____) and blood in the urine (called _hematuria_____). She was diagnosed as having a kidney infection (called _pyelonephrits_) that had developed in response to an untreated bladder infection (called_cystitis_____). Treatment included an antibiotic, force fluid, and bed rest. The development of a kidney infection from an untreated bladder infection is an example of an _ascending infection_, since the infection moved up from the bladder to the kidney. Moral of the story … do NOT ignore a bladder infection!

PART II: PUTTING IT ALL TOGETHER

MULTIPLE CHOICE

Directions. Choose the correct answer.

1. ADH
    a. is secreted by the adrenal cortex.
    b. increases the reabsorption of water from the collecting duct.
    c. is the salt-retaining hormone.
    d. increases filtration rate (GFR).

2. Why is glucose not normally found in the urine?
    a. No glucose is filtered by the glomerulus.
    b. The filtered glucose is used by the kidney cells for energy.
    c. All filtered glucose is reabsorbed.
    d. The filtered glucose is converted to creatinine and then excreted.

3. What condition is most likely to cause glucose to be excreted in the urine?
    a. hypertension
    b. renal failure
    c. hyperglycemia
    d. jaundice

4. Which of the following is least true of the urinary bladder?
    a. contains the detrusor muscle
    b. receives urine from two ureters
    c. the bladder wall is responsive to the effects of ADH
    d. micturition occurs when the detrusor muscle contracts and the internal sphincter opens

Student Name _____

5. When GFR decreases
   a. diuresis occurs.
   b. aldosterone secretion decreases.
   c. ADH secretion diminishes.
   d. urinary output declines.

6. Which of the following is a consequence of a diminished GFR?
   a. glucosuria
   b. polyuria
   c. oliguria
   d. hematuria

7. What happens at the glomerular membrane?
   a. Water and dissolved solute is filtered into Bowman's capsule.
   b. The JGA cells release ADH.
   c. The JGA cells release aldosterone.
   d. The glomerular membrane reabsorbs Na⁺.

8. Which of the following is true of the distal tubule?
   a. receives urine from the collecting duct
   b. responds to aldosterone
   c. nephron structure that is primarily concerned with filtration
   d. also called *Bowman's capsule*

9. Which of the following is not a function of aldosterone?
   a. causes Na⁺ reabsorption at the distal tubule
   b. exerts a kaliuretic effect
   c. causes the reabsorption of K⁺ by the collecting duct
   d. expands blood volume

10. Which of the following is the most accurate statement regarding creatinine?
   a. all filtered creatinine is reabsorbed
   b. no creatinine is filtered
   c. most filtered creatinine is eliminated in the urine
   d. creatinine may be secreted but is never filtered

11. An elevated serum creatinine is most indicative of
   a. cystitis.
   b. renal calculi.
   c. kidney failure.
   d. urinary retention.

12. Which of the following is a true statement?
   a. most water reabsorption occurs at the proximal tubule
   b. most filtration occurs across the walls of the collecting duct
   c. the glomerular membrane is sensitive to both ADH and aldosterone
   d. collecting duct function is regulated by ANP and BNP

13. When the renin-angiotensin-aldosterone system is activated
   a. the JGA cells secrete angiotensinogen.
   b. angiotensin I causes the adrenal cortical secretion of ADH.
   c. angiotensin II causes the adrenal cortical secretion of aldosterone.
   d. aldosterone increases the renal excretion of sodium and water.

14. Bowman's capsule receives water and dissolved solute from the
   a. proximal convoluted tubule.
   b. glomerulus.
   c. collecting duct.
   d. renal pelvis.

15. The efferent arteriole
   a. receives urine from the collecting duct.
   b. delivers blood to the peritubular capillary.
   c. delivers blood to the glomerulus for filtration.
   d. secretes converting enzyme.

16. The renal pelvis
   a. is part of the nephron unit.
   b. receives urine from the calyces.
   c. receives blood from the peritubular capillaries.
   d. concentrates the urine as it leaves the nephron unit.

17. Angiotensin II
   a. is secreted by the JGA cells.
   b. is produced in response to the activity of converting enzyme.
   c. is a powerful vasodilator.
   d. prevents the release of aldosterone.

18. Drugs (e.g., atropine) that interfere with the relaxation of the urinary bladder sphincter are most likely to cause

    a. renal failure.
    b. renal calculi.
    c. urinary retention.
    d. diuresis.

19. A person with a stenosed (narrowed) renal artery is most likely to present with

    a. urinary retention.
    b. uremia.
    c. hypertension.
    d. hematuria.

20. A person with damaged glomeruli filters large amounts of albumin and therefore develops

    a. severe hypertension.
    b. a kidney infection.
    c. edema.
    d. cystitis.

21. The development of uremia suggests

    a. a bladder infection.
    b. urinary retention.
    c. glucosuria and osmotic diuresis.
    d. renal failure.

22. Which of the following renal responses occurs when the arterial blood pressure declines to 70/50 mm Hg?

    a. The collecting duct becomes unresponsive to ADH.
    b. GFR declines.
    c. Diuresis occurs.
    d. Na^+ excretion increases.

23. Which of the following is correct?

    a. two urinary bladders
    b. two urethras
    c. two ureters
    d. one kidney

CASE STUDY

Di Uresis is a college freshman who came to the student health office complaining of pain on urination accompanied by frequency and urgency. A urine sample indicated the presence of pathogens, pus, and blood. She had no fever and no evidence of flank pain or night sweats. Polly was diagnosed as having a bladder infection. She was given an antibiotic and was instructed to force fluids and to rest.

1. Which part of the lower urinary tract was inflamed?

    a. prostate gland
    b. renal pelvis
    c. mucous membrane lining
    d. serosal lining

2. Which of the following explains why the physician was concerned that Di might develop a kidney infection?

    a. The renal artery carries infected blood to the kidney.
    b. The pathogens in the bladder can ascend (crawl up) the ureters to infect the kidneys.
    c. She might stop eating, thereby becoming more prone to infection.
    d. The high bacterial count in her urine would suppress her immune system.

3. Which of the following statements explains why bladder infections are more common in women than in men?

    a. The urethra is shorter in the female than in the male.
    b. Women excrete a less acidic urine than men.
    c. Women excrete more glucose in the urine than men.
    d. Men urinate more frequently than women.

4. Which statement about urine is true?

    a. Urine is normally colonized by *Escherichia coli.*
    b. Urinary tract infection is more common in acid urine than in alkaline urine.
    c. Urine is normally sterile.
    d. Urine normally contains glucose, protein, and pus.

PART III: CHALLENGE YOURSELF!

GROUPS AND PUZZLE

1. Which group is incorrect?

    a. tubular structures: Bowman's capsule, proximal convoluted tubule, loop of Henle, distal convoluted tubule, collecting duct
    b. hormones: ADH, aldosterone, angiotensin II
    c. "plumbing": ureters, bladder, urethra
    d. nitrogenous waste: uric acid, urea, glucose, creatinine

2. Which group is incorrect?

    a. vascular structures: glomeruli, peritubular capillaries, afferent and efferent arterioles
    b. "plumbing": ureters, bladder, nephron unit
    c. nitrogenous waste: uric acid, urea, ammonia, creatinine
    d. voluntary expulsion of urine: urination, micturition, voiding

3. Which group is incorrect?

    a. hormones: ADH, aldosterone, PTH, creatinine
    b. "plumbing": ureters, bladder, urethra
    c. nitrogenous waste: uric acid, urea, ammonia
    d. voluntary expulsion of urine: urination, micturition, voiding

PUZZLE

Hint: "Scanty and Not So Scanty"

Directions. Perform the following functions on the Sequence of Words below. When all the functions have been performed, you are left with word(s) that are related to the hint. Record your answer below.

Functions: remove the following

1. the structure across which 180 L of water is filtered/day
2. the salt-retaining hormone that is secreted by the adrenal cortex
3. the structure that contains the ascending and descending limbs
4. the name of the capillaries most concerned with reabsorption
5. the structure that is most affected by ADH
6. the cation that is excreted in response to aldosterone
7. the tube that carries urine from the renal pelvis to the bladder
8. the smooth muscle in the urinary bladder; contraction causes micturition
9. the process of urinating or voiding
10. inhibition of the reabsorption of this cation causes diuresis

Sequence of Words

ALDOSTERONEMICTURITIONPOTASSIUMGLOMERULUSLOOPOFHENLEDETRUSORO
LIGURIACOLLECTINGDUCTSODIUMPOLYURIAPERITUBULARURETERDIURESIS

Answer: Oliguria , polyuria , diuresis

Water, Electrolyte, and Acid-Base Balance

Answer Key: Textbook page references are provided as a guide for answering these questions. A complete answer key was provided for your instructor.

Objectives

1. Describe the two main fluid compartments.

2. Define intake and output.

3. List factors that affect electrolyte balance.

4. Describe the most common ions found in the intracellular and extracellular compartments.

5. List three mechanisms that regulate pH in the body.

6. Discuss acid-base imbalances: acidosis and alkalosis.

PART I: MASTERING THE BASICS

MATCHING

Fluid Compartments

Directions. Match the following terms to the most appropriate definition by writing the correct letter in the space provided. Some terms may be used more than once. See text p. 444.

A. intracellular

B. interstitial

C. plasma

D. transcellular

1. _____   water within blood vessels

2. _____   includes cerebrospinal fluid, the aqueous and vitreous humors in the eye, synovial fluids of joints, serous fluids within body cavities, and glandular secretions

3. _____   most water (about 63%) is located in this compartment

4. _____   water located between the cells

5. _____   *hypervolemia* refers to an increase in this water compartment

6. _____   also called *tissue fluid*

7. _____   largest extracellular fluid compartment

8. _____   fluid of this compartment empties into the subclavian veins

9. _____   poor skin turgor is caused by a decrease of fluid within this extracellular compartment

MATCHING

Major Ions

Directions. Match the following terms to the most appropriate definition by writing the correct letter in the space provided. Some terms may be used more than once. See text pp. 447-448.

A. sodium (Na^+)

B. potassium (K^+)

C. hydrogen (H^+)

D. bicarbonate (HCO_3^-)

E. calcium (Ca^{2+})

F. chloride (Cl^-)

1. _____   plasma concentration of this ion determines pH

2. _____   chloride usually follows the movement of this cation

3. _____   chief extracellular cation

4. _____   most diuretics work by blocking the renal reabsorption of this cation

5. _____   over 99% of this cation is stored in the bones and teeth

6. _____   neutralizes a base

7. _____   chief intracellular cation

8. _____   *hypernatremia* and *hyponatremia* refer to abnormal plasma concentrations of this ion

9. _____ *hyperkalemia* and *hypokalemia* refer to abnormal plasma concentrations of this ion

10. _____ many diuretics cause kaliuresis, thereby causing a loss of this ion

11. _____ *hypercalcemia* and *hypocalcemia* refer to abnormal plasma concentrations of this ion

12. _____ aldosterone causes the kidneys to excrete this ion

13. _____ the chief extracellular anion

14. _____ an increase in this cation causes acidosis

15. _____ regulated primarily by parathyroid hormone (PTH)

16. _____ aldosterone stimulates the kidney to reabsorb this cation

17. _____ the respiratory system is most sensitive to the plasma concentrations of this cation

18. _____ carbon dioxide (CO_2) is transported in the blood in this form

19. _____ buffers H^+

MATCHING

Acids and Bases

Directions. Match the following terms to the most appropriate definition by writing the correct letter in the space provided. The terms may be used more than once. See text pp. 448-452.

A. acidosis

B. alkalosis

1. _____ acid-base imbalance associated with a plasma pH of less than 7.35

2. _____ acid-base imbalance associated with a plasma pH of more than 7.45

3. _____ acid-base imbalance that develops when the plasma concentration of H^+ decreases

4. _____ this acid-base imbalance develops when the plasma concentration of H^+ increases

5. _____ describes an imbalance characterized by an increase in H^+ concentration and a decrease in pH

6. _____ describes an imbalance characterized by a decrease in H^+ concentration and an increase in pH

7. _____ rapid, incomplete catabolism of fatty acids produces ketone bodies and causes this acid-base imbalance

8. _____ Kussmaul respirations help correct this acid-base imbalance

9. _____ emphysema, high doses of narcotics, and splinting the chest may all cause this acid-base imbalance

10. _____ an anxious, hyperventilating patient is most likely to develop this acid-base imbalance

11. _____ any condition that causes hyperventilation causes this acid-base imbalance

12. _____ any condition that causes hypoventilation causes this acid-base imbalance

13. _____ vomiting of stomach contents is most likely to cause this acid-base imbalance

TELL A STORY

All Wet

Directions. Using the words below, fill in the blanks to complete the story. See text pp. 446-448 (also Chapter 17, pp. 306-308).

cyanosis   diuresis Na^+

K^+ dyspnea   (+) inotropic

orthopnea   water

Anna Sarca awoke suddenly at 3 AM experiencing difficulty breathing (called _____); in fact, she could only breathe when she was sitting in an upright position (called _____). Her lips were blue (called _____) and she was coughing up a pink, frothy fluid. She was rushed to the ER and was diagnosed with acute congestive heart failure and pulmonary edema. She was given digitalis to strengthen her heart (an effect called a _____ effect) and furosemide (Lasix), a "water pill." Oxygen by mask helped to relieve the respiratory distress. The furosemide acts on the renal tubules to block the reabsorption of sodium (symbol _____). As a result, _____ reabsorption is also decreased, resulting in an increase in urinary output (called _____). Unfortunately, furosemide also causes kaliuresis, the loss of _____ in the urine. Anna was soon doing better and was discharged in 1 week. Discharge medications include digitalis (Lanoxin), a thiazide diuretic, and a potassium supplement.

PART II: PUTTING IT ALL TOGETHER

MULTIPLE CHOICE

Directions. Choose the correct answer.

1. Which of the following is true of water balance?

   a. Thirst is the primary regulator of water intake.
   b. Most water is eliminated by the kidneys.
   c. Water can be lost through sensible and insensible water loss.
   d. All of the above are true.

2. What is the average adult intake of water in 24 hours?

   a. 2500 ml
   b. 500 ml
   c. 1000 ml
   d. 180 L

3. Which organ is the primary regulator of water output?

   a. lungs
   b. skin
   c. kidneys
   d. digestive tract

4. ADH

   a. is released by the posterior pituitary gland when the blood volume decreases.
   b. is the salt-retaining hormone.
   c. is a mineralocorticoid.
   d. stimulates the glomerulus to filter water.

5. Aldosterone

   a. determines the permeability of the collecting duct to water.
   b. is a neurohypophyseal hormone.
   c. stimulates the reabsorption of K^+ by the distal tubule.
   d. is the salt-retaining hormone.

6. What type of drug is most likely to cause diuresis?

   a. a drug that mimics the effects of ADH
   b. a drug that mimics the effects of aldosterone
   c. a drug that reabsorbs bicarbonate
   d. a drug that blocks the tubular reabsorption of Na^+

Student Name _____

7. Water usually follows the movement of which ion?

   a. K^+
   b. Ca^{2+}
   c. Na^+
   d. HCO_3^-

8. Poor skin turgor is

   a. indicative of blood volume expansion and heart failure.
   b. treated with antibiotics.
   c. indicative of dehydration.
   d. the earliest symptom of respiratory acidosis.

9. What does pH measure?

   a. hydration status
   b. H^+ concentration
   c. hemolysis
   d. urine concentration

10. A buffer

    a. only adds H^+.
    b. only adds bicarbonate ion.
    c. prevents changes in pH.
    d. stimulates Kussmaul respirations.

11. What is the normal range for blood pH?

    a. 7.00 to 7.35 (acid)
    b. 7.35 to 7.55 (neutral)
    c. 7.35 to 7.45 (alkaline)
    d. 6.85 to 7.45 (basic)

12. Which of the following is the first line of defense in the regulation of acid-base balance?

    a. respiratory system
    b. kidneys
    c. integumentary system
    d. buffers

13. Which of the following is not a function of aldosterone?

    a. causes Na^+ reabsorption at the distal tubule
    b. exerts a kaliuretic effect
    c. causes the reabsorption of K^+ by the collecting duct
    d. expands blood volume

14. Which of the following maintains pH by either donating H^+ or removing H^+?

    a. PTH/ADH
    b. ADH/ANF
    c. HCO_3^-/H_2CO_3
    d. Na^+/K^+

15. Why is an older adult more prone to dehydration?

    a. The collecting duct becomes overresponsive to the effects of ADH.
    b. The adrenal cortex oversecretes aldosterone.
    c. There is a decrease in the thirst mechanism.
    d. The person retains excessive sodium.

16. Which of the following systems helps correct acidosis by blowing off CO_2?

    a. renal system
    b. respiratory system
    c. baroreceptors
    d. lymphatic system

17. Why do patients in kidney failure develop acidosis? The kidneys

    a. eliminate too much water.
    b. cannot eliminate H^+.
    c. cannot eliminate K^+.
    d. make excess bicarbonate.

18. Why do patients in kidney failure become hyperkalemic? The kidneys

    a. eliminate too much water.
    b. cannot eliminate calcium.
    c. cannot eliminate K^+.
    d. fail to secrete erythropoietin.

19. In addition to buffering, how does the body of a patient in diabetic ketoacidosis try to correct the acid-base imbalance?

    a. The kidneys reabsorb all filtered H^+.
    b. The kidneys excrete bicarbonate (HCO_3^-).
    c. Rate and depth of respirations increase (Kussmaul respirations).
    d. The kidneys shut down to conserve water.

20. What does urinary specific gravity measure?

    a. the ability of the kidney to filter protein
    b. glomerular filtration rate (GFR)
    c. how much glucose is in the urine
    d. the concentration of urine

21. A kaliuretic effect is achieved when

    a. Na⁺ is reabsorbed.
    b. Ca^{2+} is excreted in the urine.
    c. blood volume expands.
    d. potassium is excreted in the urine.

22. A patient is admitted with severe emphysema and a P_{O_2} of 80 mm Hg. He has a blood pH of 7.25 and a serum bicarbonate of 40 mEq/L. Which of the following is an accurate description?

    a. metabolic acidosis and respiratory compensation
    b. metabolic alkalosis with a respiratory compensation
    c. respiratory alkalosis with a renal compensation
    d. respiratory acidosis with a renal compensation

23. Who prefers the pink end of the pH scale?

    a. Al D. O'Sterone
    b. Poly Uria
    c. Al Kalosis
    d. Hy D. Rogen

CASE STUDY

A.S. is a 65-year-old retired engineer. Five years ago he had a myocardial infarction (heart attack) and has done well since his recovery. Two days ago, he noticed that he became short of breath while walking. He is unable to sleep while lying flat and now requires three pillows. His physician determined that A.S. was in heart failure and that his lungs were "wet." He was placed on a strong diuretic, furosemide (Lasix), and digitalis (to strengthen his cardiac muscle contraction). He was also given a potassium supplement.

1. A.S.'s "wet" lungs and the inability to sleep while lying flat are indications of which condition?

    a. acidosis
    b. dehydration
    c. pulmonary edema
    d. emphysema

2. Why was the diuretic administered?

    a. remove the excess fluid
    b. strengthen the cardiac muscle contraction
    c. heal the heart muscle
    d. buffer H⁺

3. How do most diuretics work?

    a. increasing the elimination of H⁺
    b. blocking the tubular reabsorption of Na⁺
    c. making the collecting duct unresponsive to ADH
    d. decreasing the glomerular filtration of water

4. How does the heart drug digitalis increase urinary output?

    a. increases blood flow to the kidney, thereby increasing the amount of water filtered by the kidney
    b. blocks Na⁺ reabsorption by the kidney
    c. enhances the urinary excretion of K⁺
    d. antagonizes the effects of furosemide

5. Why was the potassium administered?

    a. heal the injured myocardium
    b. replace K⁺ lost because of the kaliuretic effect of the diuretic
    c. enhance the tubular reabsorption of Na⁺
    d. buffer H⁺

6. What kind of dietary modification will be prescribed?

    a. increased calcium
    b. forced fluids
    c. sodium restriction
    d. high calorie intake

PART III: CHALLENGE YOURSELF!

GROUPS AND PUZZLE

1. Which group is incorrect?

    a. cations: sodium, potassium, calcium
    b. acid-base imbalances: acidosis, alkalosis
    c. lines of defense against acid-base imbalance: buffers, lungs, kidneys
    d. transcellular fluids: aqueous humor, cerebrospinal fluid, synovial fluid, plasma

2. Which group is incorrect?

    a. transcellular fluids: aqueous humor, cerebrospinal fluid, synovial fluid
    b. buffers: bicarbonate/carbonic acid, phosphate, hemoglobin, plasma proteins
    c. lines of defense against acid-base imbalance: buffers, lungs, kidneys
    d. anions: bicarbonate, chloride, sodium

3. Which group is incorrect?

    a. cations: sodium, potassium, calcium
    b. anions: bicarbonate, chloride
    c. acid-base imbalances: acidosis, alkalosis
    d. words that relate to potassium: kaliuresis, hypokalemia, hypernatremia

PUZZLE

Hint: Who's All Wet?

Directions. Perform the following functions on the Sequence of Words below. When all the functions have been performed, you are left with word(s) that are related to the hint. Record your answer below.

Functions: remove the following

1. extracellular fluid spaces (4)

2. ions affected in hyperkalemia, hypernatremia, and hypercalcemia

3. organ that eliminates most water from the body

4. anion that follows the active pumping of sodium

5. pH imbalance caused by hypoventilation

6. any element that carries an electrical charge

7. clinical state caused by a deficiency of water

8. pH imbalance caused by vomiting stomach contents

9. NaCl → Na⁺ + Cl⁻

10. tries to maintain normal blood pH; example is $HCO_3^-/NaHCO_3$

Sequence of Words

TRANSCELLULARSODIUMKIDNEYACIDOSISANASARCACHLORIDELYMPHPOTASSIUMI
ONINTERSTITIALDEHYDRATIONIONIZATIONALKALOSISBUFFER(GENERALIZEDEDEM
A)CALCIUMPLASMA

Answer: _____, _____

Reproductive Systems

Answer Key: Textbook page references are provided as a guide for answering these questions. A complete answer key was provided for your instructor.

Objectives

1. List the structures and functions of the male and female reproductive systems.

2. Describe the structure and function of the testes.

3. Describe the structure and function of the male genital ducts.

4. Describe the accessory glands that add secretions to the semen.

5. Describe the hormonal control of male reproduction, including the effects of testosterone.

6. Describe the structure and function of the ovaries.

7. Describe the structure and function of the female genital tract.

8. Explain the hormonal control of the female reproductive cycle.

PART I: MASTERING THE BASICS

MATCHING

Reproductive Cells and Structures

Directions. Match the following terms to the most appropriate definition by writing the correct letter in the space provided. Some terms may be used more than once. See text pp. 456-459.

A. ovaries	F. seminiferous tubules	K. prepuce
B. testes	G. interstitial cells	L. external genitals
C. ovum	H. epididymis	M. scrotum
D. sperm	I. penis	N. urethra
E. spermatogonia	J. ejaculatory duct	

1. __B__   male gonads; also called *testicles*

2. __G__   cells that secrete testosterone

3. __F__   tightly coiled structures that produce sperm

4. __A__   female gonads

5. __J__   the vas deferens curves and joins with the duct of the seminal vesicle to form this duct

6. __M__   sac or pouch located between the thighs that holds the testicles

7. __B__   structure that produces sperm and secretes testosterone

8. __L__   name for the penis and the scrotum

9. __E__   undifferentiated spermatogenic cells

10. __H__   coiled structure that sits on top of the testes; a place where sperm mature

11. __N__   tubular structure that carries both urine and semen

12. __N__   tubular structure that extends from the bladder to the tip of the penis

13. __I__   male copulatory organ

14. __D__   composed of a head, body (midpiece), and tail

15. __N__   two ejaculatory ducts pass through the prostate gland and join with this urinary structure

16. __C__   female gamete

17. __K__   piece of skin that is circumcised; also called the *foreskin*

18. __D__   mature male gamete

19. __K__   skin, skin, skin, skin

Student Name _____

MATCHING

Hormones, Glands, and Semen

Directions. Match the following terms to the most appropriate definition by writing the correct letter in the space provided. See text pp. 459-461.

A. semen   E. orgasm   H. erection

B. prostate   F. impotence   I. luteinizing hormone (LH)

C. emission   G. testosterone   J. releasing hormones

D. seminal vesicles

1. __F__   the inability to achieve an erection; also called *erectile dysfunction*
2. __H__   caused by the filling of the erectile tissue by blood
3. __E__   pleasurable sensation experienced during ejaculation
4. __H__   the penis enlarges and becomes rigid
5. __G__   an androgen necessary for sperm development and for the male secondary sex characteristics
6. __C__   movement of sperm and glandular secretions from the testes and the genital ducts into the urethra
7. __J__   the hypothalamus secretes these hormones, which in turn stimulate the anterior pituitary gland to release gonadotropins
8. __B__   gland that encircles the upper part of the urethra; when enlarged, it impairs urination (dysuria)
9. __D__   gland that secretes 60% of the semen
10. __I__   also called *interstitial cell-stimulating hormone* (ICSH); stimulates the interstitial cells to secrete testosterone
11. __A__   mixture of sperm and the secretions of the accessory glands
12. __B__   donut-like gland that surrounds the upper part of the urethra as it leaves the bladder; this gland contributes to the formation of semen

ORDERING

Directions. Place these structures in order by writing the correct term in the space provided. The first one is given. See text pp. 456-459.

vas deferens   seminiferous tubules   urethra

ejaculatory duct   epididymis

1. seminiferous tubules   4. _ejaculatory duct_

2. _epididymis_   5. _urethra_

3. _vas deferens_

MATCHING

Structures of the Female Reproductive Tract

Directions. Match the following terms to the most appropriate definition by writing the correct letter in the space provided. Some terms may be used more than once. See text pp. 461-466.

A. ovaries   E. perineum   I. graafian follicle

B. oocyte   F. fallopian tubes   J. corpus albicans

C. vagina   G. follicular cells   K. hymen

D. uterus   H. corpus luteum   L. external genitals

1. __J__ the corpus luteum dies and becomes this nonsecreting structure; also known as the *white body*

2. __E__ skin-covered muscular region between the vaginal orifice and the anus

3. __D__ implantation of the embryo occurs here; also called the *womb*

4. __D__ the growing embryo and fetus live here for 9 months

5. __D__ the placenta develops in this organ

6. __F__ contains the infundibulum and fimbriae; transports the ovum to the uterus

7. __F__ fertilization occurs here

8. __D__ pear-shaped organ that is held in place by the broad ligament

9. __L__ mons pubis, labia, and clitoris; also called the *vulva*

10. __D__ parts of this organ are the fundus, body, and cervix

11. __D__ layers of this organ are the epimetrium, myometrium, and endometrium

12. __C__ 4-inch muscular tube that extends from the cervix to the vaginal opening on the perineum

13. __K__ thin membrane that partially covers the vaginal opening

14. __A__ female gonads

15. __B__ immature egg

16. __A__ target glands of FSH and LH

17. __G__ cells that surround the oocytes

18. __I__ mature ovarian follicle

19. __H__ ovarian structure that primarily secretes progesterone

20. __F__ called *oviducts* or *uterine tubes*

21. __D__ organ that has borne the entire human race

Student Name _____

MATCHING

Hormones of the Female Reproductive Cycle

Directions. Match the following terms to the most appropriate definition by writing the correct letter in the space provided. Some terms may be used more than once. See text pp. 466-469.

A. gonadotropins

B. estrogen

C. releasing hormones

D. luteinizing hormone (LH)

E. follicle-stimulating hormone (FSH)

F. progesterone

G. human chorionic gonadotropin (hCG)

1. __B__ promotes the maturation of the egg and the development of the female secondary sex characteristics

2. __F__ the "pill" contains estrogen and this hormone

3. __B__ hormone that is primarily secreted by the ovaries during the follicular phase of the ovarian cycle

4. __F__ hormone that is primarily secreted by the ovaries during the luteal phase of the ovarian cycle

5. __D__ a surge of this hormone immediately precedes ovulation

6. __F__ secreted primarily by the corpus luteum

7. __B__ a female looks female primarily because of this hormone

8. __E__ adenohypophyseal gonadotropin that acts on the ovary to stimulate the development of a follicle

9. __C__ secreted by the hypothalamus

10. __A__ classification of FSH and LH

11. __G__ hormone that stimulates the corpus luteum during early pregnancy and prevents its deterioration

12. __E__ when blood levels of estrogen and progesterone decrease at the end of the secretory phase of the uterine cycle, the anterior pituitary secretes this gonadotropin in an attempt to stimulate the development of another egg

13. __B__ ovarian hormone that dominates the proliferative phase of the uterine cycle

14. __F__ ovarian hormone that dominates the secretory phase of the uterine cycle

MATCHING

Cycles of the Female Reproductive System

Directions. Match the following terms to the most appropriate definition by writing the correct let-
ter in the space provided. Some terms may be used more than once. See text pp. 466-469.

A. ovarian cycle C. follicular phase E. ovulation

B. uterine cycle D. luteal phase F. menstrual phase

1. ___A___ composed of the follicular phase and the luteal phase

2. ___F___ also called the *period*

3. ___B___ composed of the menstrual, proliferative, and the secretory phases

4. ___C___ the ovaries primarily secrete estrogen during this phase of the ovarian cycle

5. ___D___ the ovaries primarily secrete progesterone during this phase of the ovarian cycle

6. ___E___ ejection of a mature egg at midcycle

7. ___B___ bleeding characterizes the menstrual phase of this cycle

8. ___B___ the secretory phase of this cycle is primarily due to the secretion of progesterone

9. ___B___ the proliferative phase of this cycle is primarily due to the secretion of estrogen

Student Name _____

READ THE DIAGRAM

Female Reproductive Tract

Directions. Referring to the illustration, indicate the parts of the female reproductive tract by writing the numbers on the lines provided. Some terms may be used more than once. See text pp. 461-465.

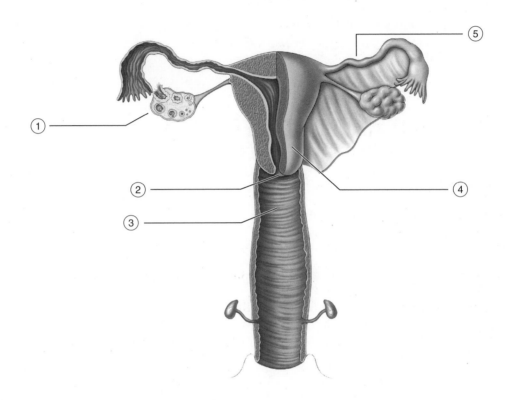

1. __4__ implantation of the embryo occurs here; also called the *womb*

2. __4__ the growing embryo and fetus live here for 9 months

3. __4__ the placenta forms in this organ

4. __5__ contains the infundibulum and fimbriae; transports the ovum to the uterus

5. __5__ fertilization occurs here

6. __4__ pear-shaped organ that is held in place by the broad ligament

7. __4__ parts of this organ are the fundus, body, and cervix

8. __4__ layers of this organ are the epimetrium, myometrium, and endometrium

9. __3__ muscular tube that extends from the cervix to the opening on the perineum

10. __1__ female gonads

11. __5__ broad ligament

12. __2__ cervix of the uterus

13. __1__ target glands of FSH and LH

14. __5__ called *oviducts* or *uterine tubes*

COLORING AND Xs AND Os

Directions. Color or mark the appropriate areas on the illustration on the previous page as indicated below.

1. Color the corpus luteum *yellow.*
2. Draw (hatched line) the path that the sperm follows to reach the egg for fertilization *blue.*
3. Place an *X* where fertilization normally occurs.
4. Place an *O* where implantation normally occurs.
5. There is a gonococcus in the vagina. Draw *arrows* showing the path that the pathogen can follow on its way to the peritoneal cavity.

PART II: PUTTING IT ALL TOGETHER

MULTIPLE CHOICE

Directions. Choose the correct answer.

1. If fertilization does not occur, the corpus luteum
   a. secretes progesterone.
   b. secretes hCG.
   c. forms the corpus albicans.
   d. forms into a placenta.

2. Ovulation
   a. normally occurs on day 14 of a 28-day cycle.
   b. is due to the secretion of hCG by the trophoblastic cells.
   c. causes the release of hormones that form the graafian follicle.
   d. normally occurs on day number 28 of a 28-day cycle.

3. When is fertilization most likely to occur?
   a. immediately after menstruation
   b. immediately before menstruation
   c. around ovulation (midcycle)
   d. day 28 of a 28-day cycle

4. With which event is the LH surge most associated?
   a. implantation
   b. ovulation
   c. ejaculation
   d. menopause

5. The luteal phase of the ovarian cycle
   a. is dominated by progesterone.
   b. requires hCG.
   c. occurs only in the pregnant state.
   d. immediately precedes ovulation.

6. The endometrium, myometrium, and perimetrium are
   a. embryonic germ layers.
   b. layers of the uterus.
   c. segments of the fallopian tubes.
   d. uterine glands that secrete the hormones of pregnancy.

7. The seminal vesicles, bulbourethral glands, and the prostate gland
   a. secrete testosterone.
   b. are called *external genitalia.*
   c. contribute to the formation of semen.
   d. are sites of sperm production.

8. What is the cause of an erection?
   a. secretion of testosterone
   b. contraction of the ejaculatory ducts
   c. filling of erectile tissue with blood
   d. emission

9. Which of the following results in sterility?
   a. phimosis
   b. circumcision
   c. vasectomy
   d. emission

10. Which of the following words best describes the reason it is necessary that the testes descend into the scrotum?

    a. temperature
    b. infection
    c. cyanosis
    d. jaundice

11. The shaft, or body, of which structure contains three columns of erectile tissue?

    a. epididymis
    b. vas deferens
    c. urethra
    d. penis

12. Which of the following is true of the process of meiosis?

    a. occurs in every cell in the body except the oocyte and spermatogonium
    b. reduces the chromosome number from 46 to 23
    c. increases the chromosome number from 23 to 46
    d. occurs in the ovum, but not the sperm

13. Which of the following is true of menopause?

    a. usually occurs in the late 20s and early 30s
    b. is always accompanied by severe and debilitating symptoms
    c. is accompanied by a gradual decrease in menstrual periods
    d. is accompanied by an increase in estrogen and progesterone secretion

14. What is the term that refers to the implantation and growth of the fetus into the walls of the fallopian tubes?

    a. menses
    b. menarche
    c. ectopic pregnancy
    d. ovulation

15. Who is most likely to grow a beard?

    a. Perry Neum
    b. Perry Metrium
    c. Tess T. O'Sterone
    d. Hy Men

CASE STUDY

K.H., an 18-year-old college student, developed strep throat. She was given an antibiotic by a physician to treat the streptococcal infection. On the following week, K.H. had no throat discomfort but began to experience an itching sensation in her vaginal area; this was accompanied by a white discharge. She purchased an over-the-counter antifungal agent and was soon symptom-free.

1. What condition did K.H. develop in response to antibiotic therapy?

    a. resistance to the antibiotic
    b. endometriosis
    c. a kidney infection
    d. a yeast infection

2. Why did this complication develop?

    a. The streptococcus had become resistant to the antibiotic.
    b. She was allergic to the antibiotic.
    c. The antibiotic had disturbed the normal flora in the vagina, thereby allowing for the overgrowth of yeast.
    d. She had taken an overdose of the antibiotic.

PART III: CHALLENGE YOURSELF!

GROUPS AND PUZZLE

1. Which group is incorrect?

    (a) parts of a sperm: head, body, corpus luteum
    b. parts of the uterus: fundus, body, cervix
    c. layers of the uterus: perimetrium, myometrium, endometrium
    d. phases of the uterine cycle: menstrual phase, proliferative phase, secretory phase

2. Which group is incorrect?

    (a) layers of the uterus: perimetrium, myometrium, cervix
    b. genital ducts: epididymis, ejaculatory ducts, vas deferens, urethra
    c. glands: seminal vesicles, bulbourethral, prostate
    d. phases of the ovarian cycle: follicular phase, luteal phase

3. Which group is incorrect?

    a. glands: seminal vesicles, bulbourethral, prostate
    (b) phases of the uterine cycle: menstrual phase, luteal phase, secretory phase
    c. gonads: ovaries, testes
    d. external genitals: penis, scrotum, labia, mons pubis

PUZZLE

Hint: "Don't Let It Die"

Directions. Perform the following functions on the Sequence of Words below. When all the functions have been performed, you are left with word(s) that are related to the hint. Record your answer below.

Functions: remove the following

1. FSH and LH
2. its midcycle surge causes ovulation
3. two ovarian hormones
4. hormone that stimulates myometrial contraction and is involved in the milk let-down reflex
5. phases of the ovarian cycle (2)
6. phases of the uterine cycle (3)
7. stimulates the breast tissue to make milk
8. site of fertilization
9. layers of the uterus

Sequence of Words

GONADOTROPINSMYOMETRIUMSECRETORYESTROGENLUTEALPROLIFERATIVEPROLAC
TINPROGESTERONELHOXYTOCINFOLLICULARMENSTRUALENDOMETRIUMHUMANCHORI
ONICGONADOTROPINFALLOPIANTUBEMAINTAINSTHECORPUSLUTEUMEPIMETRIUM

Answer: _____

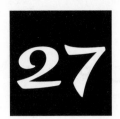

Human Development and Heredity

Answer Key: Textbook page references are provided as a guide for answering these questions. A complete answer key was provided for your instructor.

Objectives

1. Describe the process of fertilization: when, where, and how it occurs.

2. Describe the process of development: cleavage, growth, morphogenesis, and differentiation.

3. Explain the three periods of prenatal development: early embryonic, embryonic, and fetal periods.

4. State two functions of the placenta.

5. Explain hormonal changes during pregnancy.

6. Describe the hormonal changes and stages of labor.

7. Describe the structure of the breast and lactation.

8. Describe the relationships among deoxyribonucleic acid (DNA), chromosomes, and genes.

9. Explain how the sex of the child is determined.

10. State the difference between congenital and hereditary diseases.

11. Define karyotype.

PART I: MASTERING THE BASICS

MATCHING

Fertilization and Development

Directions. Match the following terms to the most appropriate definition by writing the correct letter in the space provided. Some terms may be used more than once. See text pp. 476-477.

A. fertilization

B. zygote

C. pregnancy

D. differentiation

E. cleavage

F. morphogenesis

G. development

1. _____ developmental process that refers to cell division by mitosis

2. _____ divided into trimesters

3. _____ refers to the union of the nuclei of the egg and sperm

4. _____ fertilized egg

5. _____ a cell undergoes this developmental process to become a specialized cell such as a nerve cell, muscle cell, or blood cell

6. _____ developmental process that refers to the shaping of the cell cluster

7. _____ time of prenatal development that is also called *gestation*

8. _____ also called *conception*

9. _____ process that begins with fertilization and ends with death

10. _____ a zygote-making event

MATCHING

Early Embryonic Period to Embryonic Period

Directions. Match the following terms to the most appropriate definition by writing the correct letter in the space provided. Some terms can be used more than once. See text pp. 477-483.

A. implantation

B. inner cell mass

C. morula

D. embryo

E. blastomeres

F. zygote

G. chorion

H. umbilical cord

I. amniotic fluid

J. primary germ layers

K. amniotic sac

L. blastocyst

M. extraembryonic membranes

N. placenta

1. _____ process by which the late blastocyst burrows into the endometrial lining of the uterus

2. _____ through cleavage, the zygote is transformed into this raspberry-shaped cluster of 16 cells

3. _____ cluster of cells of the blastocyst that forms the embryonic disc

4. _____ called the *bag of waters*; this bag breaks before delivery and generally signals the onset of labor

Student Name _____

5. _____ amnion, chorion, yolk sac, and allantois

6. _____ found within the amniotic sac; it forms a cushion around the embryo that helps protect it from bumps and changes in temperature

7. _____ name of baby-to-be from week 3 to week 8

8. _____ the two-cell, four-cell, and eight-cell clusters during early embryonic development

9. _____ about the fifth day, the morula becomes this

10. _____ after delivery, the stump of this structure becomes the navel, or belly button

11. _____ ectoderm, mesoderm, endoderm; all the tissues and organs of the body develop from these structures

12. _____ the outer extraembryonic membrane that forms fingerlike projections called *villi*; helps form the placenta

13. _____ this disc-shaped structure is the site where the fetal and maternal blood circulations meet; baby eats, excretes, and breathes at this site

14. _____ the hook-up or lifeline between baby and the placenta; contains blood vessels

15. _____ sperm meets egg and is called a(n) ….

READ THE DIAGRAM

Directions. Refer to Figure 27-1 in the textbook and place the following events in the correct sequence (Column 1). Indicate in Column 2 where the event takes place. See text p. 477.

late blastocyst	blastomere formation	ovulation
fertilization	implantation	early blastocyst
morula formation		

Column 1
(Ordering)

Column 2
(Location)

_____   _____

_____   _____

blastomere formation   fallopian tube

_____   _____

_____   _____

_____   _____

_____   _____

MATCHING

Fetal Period and Birth

Directions. Match the following terms to the most appropriate definition by writing the correct letter in the space provided. See text pp. 483-486.

A. fetus

B. vernix caseosa

C. colostrum

D. labor

E. parturition

F. lactation

G. lanugo

H. Braxton-Hicks contractions

I. quickening

1. _____   the developing offspring from week 9 to birth

2. _____   the experience of the mother first feeling the fetus moving during the fifth month

3. _____   the birth process

4. _____   stages are dilation, expulsion, and placental

5. _____   weak, ineffectual uterine contractions that normally occur during late pregnancy; often associated with false labor

6. _____   refers to the process of milk production

7. _____   a yellowish, watery fluid rich in protein and antibodies secreted by the mammary glands for the first 3 days following birth; baby feeds on this until the milk comes in

8. _____   a fine downy hair that covers the fetus; appears during the fifth month

9. _____   process whereby forceful contractions expel the fetus from the uterus; a response to oxytocin

10. _____   white, cheese-like substance that protects the fetus' skin from the amniotic fluid; secreted by the sebaceous glands

MATCHING

Hormones of Pregnancy

Directions. Match the following terms to the most appropriate definitions by writing the correct letter in the space provided. Some terms may be used more than once. See text pp. 478-481, 484-488.

A. human chorionic gonado-
    tropin (hCG)

B. oxytocin

C. prolactin

D. progesterone

E. aldosterone

F. parathyroid hormone
    (PTH)

1. _____   secreted by the trophoblastic cells of the blastocyst during implantation

2. _____   the placenta takes over the role of the corpus luteum and secretes estrogen and this hormone

3. _____   throughout pregnancy, this hormone inhibits uterine contractions

4. _____   thought to be responsible for morning sickness during the first trimester

5. _____   posterior pituitary hormone that stimulates uterine contractions; plays an important role in labor

6. _____ posterior pituitary hormone that plays an important role in the milk let-down reflex

7. _____ anterior pituitary hormone that stimulates the breast tissue to make milk

8. _____ hormone that is released by the adrenal cortex; it stimulates the kidneys to reabsorb Na^+ and water, thereby expanding the maternal blood volume

9. _____ hormone that keeps the maternal plasma levels of calcium high; provides baby with adequate calcium for bone growth

10. _____ the corpus luteum secretes some estrogen and larger amounts of this hormone

11. _____ secretion of this hormone continues at a high level for about 2 months, then steadily declines as the placenta takes over

12. _____ this hormone prevents deterioration of the corpus luteum

13. _____ also called *lactogenic hormone*

MATCHING

DNA, Genes, Chromosomes

Directions. Match the following terms to the most appropriate definition by writing the correct letter in the space provided. Some terms may be used more than once. See text pp. 489-492.

A. DNA
B. genes
C. chromosomes
D. autosomes
E. codominant gene

F. recessive gene
G. Down syndrome
H. mutation
I. nondisjunction
J. karyotype

K. carrier
L. dominant gene
M. sex-linked trait
N. sex chromosomes

1. _____ nucleotides that contain the base-sequencing (code) for genetic information

2. _____ DNA is tightly wound into these tightly coiled, threadlike structures

3. _____ segments of a DNA strand that carry the code for a specific trait, such as skin color or blood type

4. _____ failure of the chromosomes (or chromatids) to separate during meiosis, thereby causing the formation of eggs or sperm that have too many chromosomes

5. _____ there are 23 pairs or 46 of these in almost every human cell

6. _____ X and Y chromosomes

7. _____ genes that express a trait equally (e.g., AB blood type)

8. _____ any trait that is carried on an X or a Y chromosome

9. _____ child who has three copies of chromosome 21

10. _____ type of gene that is not expressed if it is paired with a dominant gene

11. _____ process of meiosis reduces the numbers of these by one-half (from 46 to 23)

12. _____ 22 pairs (numbered 1–22) of the chromosomes

13. _____ arrangement of chromosomes by size and shape; genetic art

14. _____ type of gene that expresses itself (e.g., brown eyes are expressed over blue eyes)

15. _____ change in the genetic code that may express itself by a change in a particular trait

16. _____ person who shows no evidence of a trait (like blue eyes) but has a recessive gene for that trait

PART II: PUTTING IT ALL TOGETHER

MULTIPLE CHOICE

Directions. Choose the correct answer.

1. Fertilization
   a. usually occurs on day 1 of a 28-day cycle.
   b. occurs within the fallopian tube.
   c. results in formation of the graafian follicle.
   d. is a direct response to FSH and LH stimulation.

2. When you were a zygote, how many cells did you have?
   a. 1
   b. 4
   c. 8
   d. 16

3. How many cells did you have when you looked most like a raspberry?
   a. 1
   b. 4
   c. 8
   d. 16

4. What is another term for a spontaneous abortion?
   a. induced abortion
   b. eclampsia
   c. placenta previa
   d. miscarriage

5. Which of the following occurs last?
   a. morula formation
   b. fertilization
   c. zygote formation
   d. implantation

6. Which of the following terms implies a genetic problem?
   a. teratogen
   b. hereditary
   c. congenital
   d. fetal alcohol syndrome

7. Which of the following conditions is most related to fetal alcohol syndrome?
   a. infection
   b. rubella
   c. teratogen
   d. heredity

8. Which of the following statements is related to the early embryonic period, the embryonic period, and the fetal period?
   a. stages of labor
   b. prenatal development
   c. first trimester of pregnancy
   d. periods of organogenesis

9. Which of the following is true of monozygotic twins?
   a. Each twin develops from a different zygote.
   b. They are fraternal twins.
   c. They are identical twins.
   d. They have congenital defects.

10. Which period involves the formation of extra-embryonic membranes, the placenta, and the period of organogenesis?
    a. period of implantation
    b. blastomere stage
    c. third trimester
    d. embryonic period

11. Which of the following is true?
    a. fertilization... ovary
    b. implantation... uterus
    c. morula formation... cervix
    d. corpus luteum... oviducts

12. Which of the following describes the organism immediately after birth?
    a. fetus
    b. embryo
    c. blastocyst
    d. neonate

Student Name _____

13. Which of the following is true of the fetal heart?

   a. the last organ to form
   b. does not become functional until the sixth month
   c. present by the second month but does not begin pumping blood until birth, when the fetal heart structures disappear
   d. pumping blood as early as the second month

14. Teratogens

   a. are fetal heart structures.
   b. cause hereditary birth defects.
   c. are always infectious agents.
   d. cause congenital defects.

15. What is the name of the effect of suckling and oxytocin release?

   a. parturition
   b. implantation
   c. the milk let-down reflex
   d. ovulation

16. Which organ or structure contains the alveolar glands and the lactiferous ducts?

   a. mammary glands
   b. pituitary gland
   c. uterus
   d. placenta

17. At birth, the extraembryonic membranes and the placenta are expelled as which structure?

   a. corpus albicans
   b. morula
   c. myometrium
   d. afterbirth

18. An oxytocic agent is one that stimulates which structure?

   a. fallopian tubes
   b. myometrium
   c. ovaries
   d. vagina

19. What is true about a child with an X and a Y chromosome? The child

   a. has Down syndrome.
   b. is male.
   c. is female.
   d. has ovaries.

20. Who will become a fetus in 8 weeks?

   a. Kary O'Type
   b. Gene
   c. Vern X. Caseosa
   d. Em B. Ryo

CASE STUDY

     P.R. has just given birth to a 7 lb baby girl and intends to breastfeed. Despite the fact that her milk has not yet come in, P.R. is encouraged to nurse her baby frequently.

1. How will the baby be nourished during the first few days? She

   a. will receive no nourishment while nursing.
   b. has no appetite and therefore will not nurse.
   c. will receive nourishment from the colostrum.
   d. will receive nourishment from bottle-feeding until her mother's milk comes in.

2. What is accomplished by frequent nursing or suckling?

   a. suppresses the secretion of prolactin
   b. stimulates lactation and the flow of milk
   c. suppresses oxytocin
   d. causes uterine bleeding

3. Which of the following hormones is necessary for lactation?

   a. insulin
   b. thymosin
   c. aldosterone
   d. prolactin

PART III: CHALLENGE YOURSELF

GROUPS AND PUZZLE

1. Which group is incorrect?

    a. extraembryonic membranes: amnion, chorion, yolk sac, allantois
    b. primary germ layers: ectoderm, mesoderm, endoderm
    c. embryonic structures: zygote, blastomere, morula, blastocyst, fetus
    d. genes: dominant, recessive, codominant

2. Which group is incorrect?

    a. embryonic structures: zygote, blastomere, morula, blastocyst
    b. hormones: estrogen, progesterone, hCG, prolactin, oxytocin
    c. genetic disorders: Down syndrome, Edward's syndrome, eclampsia
    d. stages of labor: dilation, expulsion, placental

3. Which group is incorrect?

    a. genes: dominant, recessive, codominant
    b. genetic disorders: Down syndrome, Edward's syndrome, Patau's syndrome
    c. stages of labor: dilation, expulsion, proliferative
    d. ovarian structures: corpus luteum, corpus albicans, graafian follicle

PUZZLE

Hint: "A Zygoting Event"

Directions. Perform the following functions on the Sequence of Words below. When all the functions have been performed, you are left with word(s) that are related to the hint. Record your answer below.

Functions: remove the following

1. structure in which fertilization normally occurs
2. organ in which implantation normally occurs
3. distal neck-like region of the uterus
4. muscle layer of the uterus
5. cells that secrete hCG
6. top dome-shaped part of the uterus
7. this gland also serves as the site where the fetus breathes, eats, and excretes
8. fluid in which the fetus is immersed
9. extraembryonic membranes (4)
10. a virus or drug that is capable of causing a monsterlike congenital defect
11. three primary germ layers
12. baby is covered in white cream cheese
13. organ that produces the mature ovum
14. the blastomere gives rise to this raspberry
15. types of twins

Sequence of Words

FALLOPIANTUBEOVARYMESODERMAMNIONPLACENTAAMNIOTICFUNDUSCHORIONENDO
DERMMYOMETRIUMTROPHOBLASTICCELLSYOLKSACDIZYGOTICVERNIXCASEOSACERVIXUT
ERUSTERATOGENECTODERMMONOZYGOTICALLANTOISFERTILIZATIONMORULA

Answer: _____